BEAUTY
FROM THE
INSIDE OUT

BEAUTY FROM THE INSIDE OUT

DIANA BIHOVA, M.D.

AND CONNIE SCHRADER

RAWSON ASSOCIATES
NEW YORK

Library of Congress Cataloging-in-Publication Data
Bihova, Diana.
Beauty from the inside out.
Includes index.
1. Beauty, Personal.   2. Women—Health and Hygiene.
I. Schrader, Constance, 1933–   II. Title.
RA778.B55   1987   646.7'042   84-42927
ISBN 0-89256-282-X

Published simultaneously in Canada by Collier Macmillan Canada, Inc.

Copy edited by Bob Oskam

Packaged by Rapid Transcript, a division of March Tenth, Inc.
Composition by Folio Graphics
Printed and bound by Fairfield Graphics, Fairfield, Pennsylvania
Designed by Jacques Chazaud

First Edition

To my inspiration,
my beautiful daughter,
Jennifer

CONTENTS

ACKNOWLEDGMENTS

I am grateful to my publisher, Eleanor Rawson, for seeing the merit in this project long before it was a finished book.

I would like to thank Susan Cohen for believing in the project and for her moral support and Audrey Liounis for her editorial guidance.

A special note of gratitude goes to Rosamond Bernier and John Russell for their encouragement and helpful suggestions.

Those dermatologists who have been involved in my training and my career deserve my warmest thanks: Dr. Allan Shalita, chairman of the Department of Dermatology at Downstate Medical Center, for giving me the opportunity to fulfill my dream of becoming a dermatologist; and Dr. Rudolf Baer, former chief of the Skin and Cancer Unit at New York University Medical Center, for giving me the chance to be affiliated with this wonderful department.

And, finally, I would like to offer my sincere thanks to all my patients, who inspired this book.

Connie Schrader is deeply grateful to Eugene Winick, Esq., and Suzanne Lorenzo for their wisdom, patience, and help; to Ernst-Joseph Schrader, Jr., for his midnight work; to Kathie Gordon for her support and help; and to Jean Brown, Irma Heldman, and Gloria Mosseson for their interest and friendship.

BEAUTY FROM THE INSIDE OUT

BEFORE YOU BEGIN
THIS BOOK . . .

Women are different. This book is written primarily for women and focuses on those differences. I've tried to answer the questions my patients and friends often ask and also to address some of those that aren't asked but are usually surrounded by misinformation.

The time has come for women to look at beauty from a more scientific point of view. Beauty is indeed "more than skin deep." *Beauty from the Inside Out* explains how fundamental biological processes affect your skin, hair, and nails, and I hope the information here will make it possible for you to work in harmony with your unique heredity and biology to improve your appearance.

I have tried to go into as much depth as possible to explain the *whys* as well as the *whats* of personal care. I have also tried to help you find realistic solutions to your personal beauty needs amidst the clouds of speculation, advertising, and misinformation.

This is not a dermatological textbook, nor is it a beauty book in the traditional sense. I have presented some of the frustrating skin and hair problems you may face, as well as tips on improving your appearance. Several of the chapters are organized around life-style activities, because your skin and hair go everywhere with you—they are your introduction to the world. They can also be affected by everything in and around you.

While science has given women a new potential for beauty, society has made life ever busy, hyperactive, and harried. My hope is that *Beauty from the Inside Out* will give you the information you want and need to look your best in spite of today's pressures. We all want to look and feel our best, and I hope that my insights as a woman dermatologist will help you achieve that.

1

YOUR PERFECT

PACKAGING

My interest in skin must have started the first time I recognized myself in the mirror. I can't remember when I wasn't aware of how I looked, and how other people looked.

Your skin keeps you in and the outside out. It is what people see when they look at you. In just a fleeting glance, your personal banner—your skin and how healthy, cared for, and firm it is—tells the world who you are: your general age, and more than you might want to reveal about how you think and what you think of yourself.

Your skin is strong, tough, delicate, and fragile.

What Your Skin Does Every Day

Your skin is:

- A shield protecting internal organs against mechanical and radiation damage and invasion by foreign substances and organisms
- The house of many sense organs, allowing you both to react to danger and enjoy pleasure
- A regulator that keeps your internal temperature stable
- A storehouse for needed nutrients
- An excretory organ, helping to eliminate waste products

If you are of average size, the surface area of your skin is about 3,000 square inches (as large as a dining table) and weighs approximately six pounds (twice as much as the three-pound brain). The 10 percent of the total skin that is on the face and head makes a big difference in what others think about you and what you think about yourself. In a single square inch of your

5

cheek, there are approximately 20 blood vessels, 65 hairs, 100 or more oil glands, 650 or more sweat glands, 28 nerves, 13 sense receptors for cold, 78 for heat, and 1,300 for pain.

Layers of Skin

Your skin is made of three different types of tissue. The outer skin layer, the epidermis, is partly composed of dead tissue; the inner, thicker layer, the dermis, consists of dense connective tissue. The two layers are not flat surfaces cemented together. They fit in a series of grooves. Fatty tissue makes up the third, or subcutaneous, layer.

Each layer varies in thickness; the thinnest skin of the body is on the eyelids. For most women, the thickest skin is on the soles of the feet.

The epidermis and the dermis each are divided into several layers. Bundles of collagenous (protein) tissue extend downward from the dermis to anchor the skin firmly onto the underlying tissue.

Nutrients from the food you eat, water, and oxygen are transferred upward to the epidermis. Several specialized groups of cells form into sweat and oil glands, hair and nails, and sometimes into skin growths such as moles.

Epidermis

Not all of your skin is seen. The part that people recognize is the epidermis, the outermost layer. The epidermis can be smooth and soft or rough and dry. The epidermis itself is composed of several layers of cells; the outermost of these is made up of dead skin cells and is called the horny layer. This is the barrier that your skin presents to the outside world; its cells are keratinized (hard and horny).

These flat, horny cells are about 80 percent protein and only about 20 percent water (compared with about 70 percent water for internal living cells). The thickness of this layer varies. Men have a thicker top layer than women have.

The keratin of the horny layer fairly effectively waterproofs the skin. The acidity, or pH, of the cells in the layer also helps to destroy certain microorganisms. Healthy dry skin is naturally antibacterial.

The deepest layer of the epidermis is subdivided into a spinous layer and, beneath it, a basal layer. The cells of this basal layer multiply and endlessly reproduce to replace the worn and used cells of the horny layer. It is this continuous reproduction of skin that allows you to peel, heal, and still have skin.

Skin cells live an average of twenty-four to thirty days, but the replacement rate of dead skin cells at the outer surface varies immensely. For example, the elbow's outer layer is replaced every ten days; the knee's every twenty days; and the forearm crook's every hundred days.

Some of the cells in the basal layer's skin reproduction factory are melanocytes. These specialized cells create granules of melanin, a natural brown-black pigment that gives the skin its color. Everyone, regardless of skin color or sex, has the same number of melanocytes. The size of the granules and the amount of pigment they produce are genetically determined and vary from person to person. Melanin is your skin's natural sunscreen. It is a protection against the sun's ultraviolet rays. (The pinkish tone of very fair skin is really an absence of skin color plus the showing through of blood vessels in the underlying dermis. Yellow tones of the skin are provided by carotene found in the horny layer and in the fatty regions below the dermis.)

Your skin is like no one else's in the world—even if you have an identical twin—because of its unique pattern of whorls, arches, and loops in the epidermal surface of your fingertips and palms.

Dermis

The dermis is your true skin. It is a dense layer of connective tissue containing white collagenous fibers, some yellow elastic fibers, and others. Blood, lymph vessels, nerves, hair follicles, and sweat and sebaceous glands are embedded in the dermis. The reproductive layer of the epidermis is nourished through the dermis.

The dermis nourishes the basal layer of the epidermis. It is also attached to the lower layer of subcutaneous fat by a fibrous network of connective tissue that makes the skin tough, moveable, and elastic. Most movements of the body require some stretching or wrinkling of the skin, and the structure of the dermis is what makes that possible. However, even young skin has limited elasticity. When stretched too far, as in pregnancy or extreme weight gain in a short period of time, tiny tears may occur. We see them as stretch marks.

The Secret of Young Skin

To keep your skin looking young, you must keep your dermis full, soft, and elastic. You must also keep your epidermis smooth and moist. I'm going to discuss many agents and activities that improve or harm the skin, but one factor towers over all the others in the way it affects the skin—the sun.

Excessive exposure to the sun makes the dermis thin and inelastic and the epidermis dry, rough, and dull. Think about the irony of this as you struggle to improve your skin in order to flaunt it on the sunny beach!

Blood and Lymphatic Vessels

Embarrassment can make you blush, fear can make you pale, and anger can turn you either hot or cold. Emotions affect the skin's supply of blood. Networks of blood vessels in the dermis and around the hair follicles and the sweat and oil glands usually keep the skin warm and rosy in tone.

When your skin's blood vessels are all distended, as on a hot day, there is a cooling effect on the surface of your skin due to heat loss. Constriction of the vessels limits the flow of the blood to the skin either to conserve body heat or as part of the body's stress-fighting mechanism. (Blood diverted from the skin provides an additional supply for the brain, heart, and muscles, which may be called on for flight or fight to cope with an impending emergency.)

Besides a complex network of blood vessels, your skin has a complex network of lymphatic vessels that form a communication system and transport fluids.

Subcutaneous Tissue—Getting Under Your Skin

Your dermis is attached to underlying fat by strong tissue sheets that actually are bundles of collagen. The boundary between the dermis and this fat layer is not sharply defined, and even hair follicles are sometimes found in this layer.

Subcutaneous fat is unevenly distributed. Some areas, such as the thighs, tend to have heavy layers of fat; other areas, such as the eyelids and male genitalia, have very little. The layers of fat act as heat insulators and shock absorbers.

For Women Only: Cellulite

If you are a woman, the connective tissue between the dermis and fat is vertical. In men this connective tissue is almost horizontal. With this vertical arrangement of tissue, an increase in the body's fat cells coupled with a weakening of the dermis can lead to protrusions of the subcutaneous tissue's fat compartments into the lower part of the dermis. When this protrusion occurs it creates a granular texture sometimes called "the mattress phenomenon" but more often called "cellulite." Since only women have vertical connective tissue, only women have cellulite. Blame it on your hormones.

Some cellulite therapy employs injections of enzymes to destroy fat tissue. But the most logical, least painful, and most obvious way to rid yourself of cellulite is to rid yourself of excessive fat deposits. A low-fat diet, regular exercise, and avoidance of high-salt foods (edema caused by water retention affects the dermis) usually work to reduce cellulite. But they work slowly. In the long run, weight loss is most effective.

Absorption

Can skin creams penetrate your skin, or is it all copywriting?

At one time human skin was thought to be an almost impenetrable barrier. Even chemists and physicians believed that paints and cosmetics applied to the skin could not be absorbed. Now we know that many chemicals can be absorbed and that gases and some oils pass through the skin with relative ease.

Vitamins A, D, and K and a variety of hormones are all absorbed by the skin. The salts of mercury, arsenic, lead, tin, copper, and bismuth, when combined with sebum, the skin's oil, acquire the ability to penetrate the skin. (Nearly all these poisonous salts were used at one time or another in cosmetics—with disastrous, life-threatening results.)

Happily, carbon monoxide will not penetrate the skin, while oxygen (and many other gases) will. There is some evidence that absorption of oxygen into the skin and release of carbon dioxide from it (the quantities involved are small) contribute to your skin's health.

Most of the barrier effect that your skin has is based on electrical or ionic interactions between the horny and other layers of skin.

Nerves and Sense Organs

Close your eyes and run your fingers over this page. Your fingers will give you a fairly detailed picture of the paper: dry, slightly rough, rectangular in shape. You can sense its relative weight and whether or not it is stiff.

The skin is one of the brain's most important sources of information. Messages continuously flow back and forth between the skin and the central nervous system. Certain areas—the lips, the nipples, and the fingertips, for example—are lavishly supplied with sense receptors, while other areas, such as the small of the back, have fewer. The density of these sense receptors is important for working—and loving.

If you lose feeling in an area of the skin as a result of injury or frostbite, it is very serious. Then you must watch yourself constantly to avoid hurting yourself without knowing it.

Your Thermostat

On a cold, wintry day the difference in temperature between your inner self and the outer world can be as much as 100°F. Your skin is your body's insulator and regulator.

Your outer skin is most comfortable at about 70°F, while the inner body must maintain a temperature of about 98°F. What accounts for this disparity between inner and outer temperatures is that heat is continuously produced as a by-product of muscle contractions and the various chemical reactions of cell metabolism. You've probably noticed that exercise, which uses muscles, and eating a large meal, which requires a surge of metabolic activity (the chemical action of turning food into cell nutrients), both make you warmer.

The skin's surface acts as a radiator. Body heat is carried by the blood through the abundant skin capillaries to the dermis, and radiates away. The skin's continuous secretion of perspiration also carries substantial heat to the surface of the skin, and evaporating perspiration adds another form of cooling to the system. (The movement of air in the form of a breeze makes cooling go faster.)

When the air around you is cold, heat retention is necessary. Then the muscular walls of the skin's blood vessels constrict and reduce the blood flow to the skin's surface. Minute muscles around each hair tighten, erecting the hairs and forming bumps (goose bumps); large muscles tighten, causing shivering, which also creates heat. The skin automatically keeps the body's internal temperature constant despite variations in the temperature of the skin.

Sebaceous Glands—Oily Skin/Dry Skin

Except for a few areas such as the soles of the feet and the palms of the hands, the entire body is covered with hair follicles. Even the most seemingly hairless woman or child is covered with a myriad of tiny follicles and soft, fine hair.

Clustered around each hair follicle are several sebaceous (oil) glands— microscopic, bulblike formations. In a few regions of the skin, such as the eyelids, oil glands open directly onto the surface of the skin rather than into the hair follicles.

Sebaceous glands vary greatly in size and density; those in the face, back, and chest are very large and numerous compared with those in other areas. (Note that the face, back, and chest are also the areas most prone to acne.) The sebaceous glands secrete an oily substance called sebum, which contains fats, cell debris, and salts. One type of fat in sebum, known as triglyceride, is similar to the fat found in meat and provides an irresistible feast for bacteria.

Sebum is an important element in the skin's system of keeping itself clean and protected. As it flows out from the follicles it brings waste products with it and prevents foreign particles from entering the pores. It also coats the surface of the skin with a slightly acidic, protective oily film that keeps the outer skin and hair from becoming dry and inflexible.

When the temperature rises and the pores—the visible openings of the follicles on the skin's surface—open to allow more skin evaporation and cooling, more sebum is exuded than usual. When the temperature falls, the tiny muscles around the follicles tighten and shut down sebum production. That is why skin seems oilier in hot weather than in cool weather.

Oil glands slow with age. The secretion of the sebaceous glands is controlled by male sex hormones, or androgens, which both men and women have. Sebaceous glands are the most sensitive androgen organs in our bodies. At puberty, late in pregnancy, or when you are under stress, there is a spurt of glandular activity caused by elevated levels of male hormones; the production of sebum noticeably increases. In adolescence this effect is expected, but it can and does happen at other times. Despite many ups and downs, however, hormone levels tend to fall as you age, resulting in less active sebaceous glands. Thus dry skin is usually a problem of older skin.

You Are Your Skin

Lovely skin is almost synonymous with human beauty. The art and science of skin care consist of working with the skin, not against it, to heal or diminish the blemishes that afflict it while highlighting its natural tone and texture. Skin requires tender loving care, and to give that—while avoiding the temptations of faddish but harmful practices—you need to keep the skin's basic structure in mind.

2

KEEPING YOUR SKIN YOUNG AND MOIST

Dry skin is an epidemic across the land. Each year from November through April I see patients who suffer itching and chapping. I also see patients who struggle year round with the rough texture of dry skin. Some patients in their teens or barely in their twenties already show signs of wrinkling.

Although pharmaceutical companies produce thousands of dry skin lotions, ointments, and creams, dry skin remains a major problem. Why does it happen, and what is the best way to keep skin smooth and soft—and youthful?

What Is Dry Skin?

The outermost layer of the epidermis normally protects human skin against the loss of moisture. When too much moisture escapes, skin becomes dry, red, and irritated.

These factors dry the skin by stripping away protective oils or by increasing evaporation of moisture (water) from your skin's surface:

- Exposure to sun
- Harsh soaps or incorrect cleansing
- Strong winds
- Low temperatures
- Low humidities
- Repeated wetting and drying
- Heating systems that cause dry air
- Air conditioners
- Saunas
- Overly long or hot baths
- Rough or tight clothing
- Poor nutrition

If you or your close relatives have hay fever, asthma, or very dry skin, you may have inherited what is called an atopic background and be extremely prone to skin dryness.

Water is one of the substances that can soften skin naturally. Human skin is most comfortable, smooth, and healthy when its outer layers are about 10 to 20 percent water. When the humidity in the air around you is 70 percent, the moisture in the outer layer of your skin will be about 10 percent water. If the relative humidity in the surrounding air decreases (as it does in winter, because cold air cannot hold as much moisture as warm air), the moisture level in the skin's outer layer drops.

When there isn't enough moisture, the surface of the skin begins to shrink and crack. When it dries, it becomes hard and brittle. The more cracked the skin is, the less effective it is as a guard against the outside environment. Have you ever noticed that when you apply a moisturizer there is sometimes a slight stinging sensation on very chapped knees or hands? Your skin is so sensitive that it is reacting to the chemicals in the moisturizer. (Never let your skin get that chapped!) Cracks allow bacteria to enter and your skin becomes infected, tender, and vulnerable.

Not all the moisture in the skin's outer layer comes from the air; some comes from the dermis beneath the outer layers of the skin. But the upward movement of the moisture to the outer layers is slow and insufficient. Because of this, efforts to remoisturize dehydrated skin solely from within are doomed to fail.

For example, if you applied a thick layer of petroleum jelly to your skin to prevent moisture from escaping and then drank a large quantity of water in the hope that the water would pass through the bloodstream to the dermis and from there moisturize the top layer of skin, you'd be disappointed. It wouldn't work. The most effective way to deal with dry skin is at the surface of the skin itself.

Do You Have Dry Skin—Without Knowing It?

- Does your skin feel tight or itchy after washing?
- Does your skin look dull?
- Does your skin feel rough?
- Are you bothered by tiny lines around your eyes?
- Does your skin often feel raw, tender, and sore, and is it red sometimes?

If you have answered yes to even two of these questions, you probably have dry skin in some areas of your face. You are not alone.

Dry skin begins in subtle ways. The first signs are scaliness and roughness, followed by small fissures or cracks in the skin (chapped areas). The cracks usually appear red and may even bleed.

When your skin becomes dry, the usually invisible particles of mature skin cells clump together and shed in large flakes or scales that peel off, leaving behind red and sensitive skin. The flakes dropping off can easily be seen against dark clothing. When scaling is severe it exposes the deeper layers of skin beneath the damaged horny layer. Itching follows and often an itch/scratch cycle develops that is hard to stop.

Age is a contributing factor. With age the skin cells weaken and skin loses the ability to hold moisture. Decreased oil production also plays a role. Patches of dry skin appear: The legs, arms, throat, eye area, and backs of the hands show dryness first. But dryness can strike anyone, at any time. It can sometimes be associated with other health problems such as asthma and hay fever.

Three Steps to Putting Moisture Back in Your Skin

Dry skin can be controlled. Preventive measures can inhibit moisture loss and control those conditions that aggravate the skin and contribute to dryness.

Since dry skin is actually the loss of moisture, it would seem logical that applying water to chapped areas would soothe them and solve the problem. This isn't the way it works; simply applying water to the skin is not a good way to rehydrate. The skin's surface has been damaged and it cannot retain moisture unless those tiny droplets are held in place on the skin. Placing water on dry skin without holding it in place will encourage evaporation and actually make the skin drier.

Here is the best way to remoisturize dry skin:

1. Soak the dry area in moderately warm water for ten minutes. If the area is on the face, immerse your face in warm water while breathing through a straw, or gently steam your skin by making a tent of a towel and holding your face near hot—not boiling—water.
2. Gently blot your skin with an absorbent terrycloth towel. Remove only dripping water; you will want some moisture left on the skin surface.
3. Immediately coat the skin with moisturizer to seal water.

Many excellent hydrating products—such as lanolin and petroleum jelly—are thick and oily. (Eucerin Moisturizing Formula is one such product.) These are usually oils to which some water has been added, and they are called water-in-oil emulsions. Water in oil tends to block evaporation, but a blocking product is useless if it is applied before the skin is soaked and moistened.

If you find your skin dry, tight, and chapped, immediately applying a thick coat of cream will not help as much as applying the cream after the skin has been moisturized with water. I always apply moisturizer directly after my bath or shower because this is when moisturizer penetrates deeper and more easily. You can also touch your face with a warm, wet towel before applying moisturizer. Placing plastic film or Saran Wrap over very dry areas such as legs or arms (not the face) after moisturizing with oily products enhances effectiveness of the products.

Avoid thin, watery products if your skin is very dry. They usually are oil-in-water emulsions (more water than oil). When these are applied to the skin the water in the product evaporates, making the skin feel cool. The evaporation does nothing to help dry skin.

Which Moisturizer Should You Use?

Degrees of Dryness	*Moisturizer*
Mild—your skin feels taut after washing. It is often scaly and rough.	Keri Lotion (Westwood) Neutrogena Moisture (Neutrogena) Lubriderm Lotion (Warner-Lambert) Nutribel (Lancôme) Aquacare Dry Skin Cream and Lotion (Herbert)
Moderate—your skin has pronounced scaliness and roughness and becomes irritated easily. After bathing it chaps, cracks, and sometimes itches.	Complex 15 Cream (Baker/Cummins) LactiCare Lotion (Stiefel) Aquacare/HP Dry Skin Cream and Lotion (Herbert) Purpose Cream (Ortho) Carmol 10 Lotion (Syntex)
Severe—your skin is red, sore, and itchy most of the time. Small, painful cracks may bleed and become infected. *See a dermatologist as soon as possible.*	Carmol 20 Cream (Syntex) Ultra Mide 25 Lotion (Baker/Cummins) Lac-Hydrin (Westwood)—by prescription only

Moisturizers for Those Allergic to Fragrances or Lanolin

- Moisturel (Westwood)—fragrance-free
- Dramatically Different Moisturizing Lotion (Clinique)—fragrance-free
- Nutraderm (Owen)—lanolin-free

Miracle Products?

If you are like most of us, you will use any product that promises relief when your skin feels itchy, parched, and uncomfortable. Promises are never lacking; there are always new products on the market that claim to duplicate the skin's natural lubricating oils and to keep the skin smooth and youthful. A product is "miraculous" only if it works for you.

Many products contain vegetable oils—for example, oils derived from avocados, apricot kernels, jojoba beans, or most recently, the sap of the aloe vera plant. Still other products contain animal oils—turtle oil, mink oil, and sheep oil (sheep oil is lanolin, a wonderful substance, except that many women are allergic to it) are the most common. Products that contain mysterious substances from beautiful plants and healthy, glossy-coated animals have psychological appeal but are little more than standard water-in-oil mixtures. If you are allergic to any of them, any one of these so-called miracle oils can create a problem.

Creams and lotions that contain elastin, collagen, and other natural proteins of the skin often are very expensive. But in tests they perform only slightly better than the standard water-in-oil preparations. (For more on collagen and elastin, see chapter 8).

Moisturizers containing essential fatty acids have been found to be quite effective.

Natural Moisturizing Factor

Many products are described as containing "natural moisturizing factor" (NMF) similar to the natural moisturizers in the horny layer of the skin. These products do seem to aid the skin's ability to absorb and retain moisture in its upper layers. It is believed that NMF either binds the water to hold it in place or keeps the keratin organized so that it can more readily become hydrated.

Ingredients That Work to Soften and Smooth Skin

Lactic acid when used in a 2 to 5 percent concentration seems to enhance your skin's ability to hold moisture. (In higher concentrations it has a tendency to loosen the epidermal cells of the skin and cause flaking.)

Allantoin, a colorless crystal that is soluble in hot water and prepared chemically from uric acid, seems to soften and soothe skin. It is thought that allantoin may disrupt the skin's structure, leading to greater penetration of water and more rapid and better moisturizing. The substance is in creams that are rubbed into the skin. It must be applied before the skin is soaked in water, and then followed by an emollient after the soaking.

Glycerine is a by-product of the manufacture of soap. It has been used as a skin moisturizer for hundreds of years. It attracts moisture from both the environment and the underlying dermal layer of skin. Glycerine and rose water solutions, in equal proportions, were once the only hand creams "ladies" used. Glycerine is most effective in very humid places, since there must be moisture in the atmosphere for it to attract. Beware of any product that contains glycerine if your skin is dry and you are in a cold or dry climate: It will just speed chapping because it will draw moisture out of your tissues.

Urea, used by the ancients in beauty preparations, has been included in many commercial products since the 1940s. It is safe and effective in concentrations of 2 to 25 percent. Urea binds to the skin's natural protein and encourages flaking of dead cells. Because of this, urea aids in the removal of scales and crusts and enhances water uptake into the skin's outer layer. Some urea-based moisturizers are:

- Carmol 10 Lotion (Syntex)
- Carmol 20 Cream (Syntex)
- Nutraplus Lotion and Cream (Owen)
- Aquacare/HP Dry Skin Lotion and Cream (Herbert)
- Ultra Mide 25 Moisturizer Lotion (Baker/Cummins)

Ten Ways to Beat Dry Skin

1. Avoid strong winds and sunbathing.
2. Humidify your home or work area. (Buy a humidifier or place pans of water near heating sources.)
3. Avoid frequent long, leisurely bubble baths and long showers.
4. Don't use harsh soaps or detergents.
5. Avoid saunas and apply a moisturizing lotion to your skin directly after you use a steam bath.
6. Blot your skin after bathing; apply moisturizer over still damp skin.
7. Keep away from chemical irritants. Wear cotton-lined rubber gloves when you have to do piles of dishes or hand laundry with detergents. Solvents of all kinds play havoc with your skin.
8. Wear soft, smooth, silky clothing; don't wear rough woolens and linens next to your skin. If you like a tweedy look, cover your skin with a soft cotton undershirt or T-shirt. Don't wear excessively tight clothes that rub against your skin.
9. Wear protective gloves, scarves, and even sunglasses to prevent your skin from becoming dehydrated through exposure to wind.
10. Be sure your diet includes sufficient vitamin A (yellow vegetables, fish, liver, milk, and margarine) and vitamin E (vegetable oils, liver, leafy green vegetables, whole grains).

(To learn more about diet and your skin, see chapter 17.)

What Is the Best Treatment for Dry Skin?

What is the best product? Whatever product suits you best in texture, form, and effectiveness is best for you. And remember: No dry skin product will work unless you use it—often.

Lotions and creams are favorites because they are washable and can be rubbed into the skin so they are almost invisible. But they are also nonocclusive—too thin to stop much evaporation.

Ointments resist removal and are messy. Thick, gooey products with an ointment base are most effective, but they stain clothing and bed linens. If you are like me and can't stand the mess, try to confine ointments to small, severely chapped areas such as the backs of the hands, the throat, and perhaps the eye area.

Fast-drying gels should be avoided because they have a high alcoholic content. If you feel any cooling sensation after applying a lotion or gel, you know that evaporation is taking place and that you will soon be drier than before.

How to Wash Dry Skin

If you suffer from dry skin, avoid washing unnecessarily. When you do wash use lukewarm water and avoid alkaline soaps, which tend to strip all surface oils from your skin. The following soaps will do the least damage:

Superfatted Soaps	*"Soapless" Soaps*
Oilatum Soap (Stiefel)	Emulave Bar (Cooper)
Derma Soap (Derma)	Lowila Cake (Westwood)
Basis Extra Dry Skin Soap (Beiersdorf)	
Neutrogena Dry Skin Soap (Neutrogena)	

Keep the lather centered on the back and shoulders and other oily areas of the body, such as around the groin. It's not necessary to use soap on your legs and arms daily. I do not recommend using any type of soap on the face. (For how to clean the skin of your face if it tends to be dry, see chapter 3.)

How to Take a Nondrying Bath

Baths may help you relax, but they can also dry your skin. Here are some ways to make sure your leisurely bath won't ruin your skin:

- Limit baths to a maximum of three per week.
- Try using shower and bath gels, such as Neutrogena Rainbath, instead of soap.
- Always use lukewarm—never hot—water.
- Bathe at night rather than in the morning. Your skin develops natural oils during the day.
- Add bath oils after you've soaked in the bath for at least five minutes. The soaking will plump up your outermost skin cells, then the oil can

seal the moisture onto your skin. Bath oils can also be applied directly to dry skin in the shower.

Overnight Creams

A flip through the pages of a woman's magazine or a walk through a department store's cosmetics section will introduce you to so-called skin-renewal or cell-repair creams. These are the latest efforts of cosmetic chemists to help your skin help itself.

Most claim to speed the turnover of skin cells so that old cells on the surface of the skin are shed faster. The new creams may actually do this. However, claims that hormone-containing creams will retard aging or make skin look younger are misleading. The negligible amounts in which hormones are present cannot possibly change skin functions.

Pumice, clarifiers, and exfoliants work on the same premise. Improvement in the skin's tone and texture is a natural concomitant to fresher cells on its surface.

Young Skin—How to Have It

The only sure way of slowing the arrival of aging skin is to avoid all exposure to ultraviolet rays and to use the facial muscles as little as possible. This would mean no laughing, no talking, and never seeing the light of day. More realistically, proper skin care involves understanding how your skin works and using the right moisturizers and sunscreens to protect it. And remember that sleep is the best overnight restorer.

3

START CLEAN

I don't remember when I first started to wash my own face—and you probably don't either. Think how many times you've washed or cleansed your skin. It is the most basic of all skin care treatments and to me one of the most important. Before I use any cleanser, I want to know if it is right for my skin. Trial and error is the way most people select a cleanser, but you can do better if you know something about the benefits and drawbacks of each product and how the products should be used.

Make Mine Cleanser

I am not a soap user. This is not because I have sensitive skin (in fact, I have combination skin) but because I find that all soaps, even superfatted ones, dry the skin. Even if your skin doesn't get red or scaly, if your face feels tight after you wash it, the soap is having a drying effect.

I prefer instead to wash my face with a mild cleanser (some good ones are Cetaphil Lotion from Owen, Skin Sense from Molton Brown, and Neutrogena's) twice a day—in the morning and at night. Another part of my cleansing routine involves using a brush similar to a man's shaving brush, or a sea sponge, on my face every other day to lightly exfoliate the surface and get my circulation going.

As a dermatologist I can say that many of the skin problems I have seen stem from the soaps my patients use. Soap is still the standard because it is inexpensive, reliable, easy to use, and wonderful for the rest of your body. Soap is an emulsifying agent, able to attach itself both to water molecules and to oil and dirt molecules from the skin, pulling them together in an emulsion (mixture) and allowing them to be rinsed away easily. It is composed of sodium and potassium salts produced by the action of alkali on fatty acids such as coconut oil and tallow. It can be made from olive oil, lard, or any fatty substance, but additives or a greater proportion of some ingredients give a brand or type of soap its special texture or properties.

Skin and Soap

Human skin is slightly acidic, with a pH usually between 5.5 and 6.5. Most soaps are alkaline substances; the alkali strips the skin of its outer oily layer as it strips the dirt. The natural pH of the skin is altered very slightly after washing, but within two or three hours the acidic oils from the oil glands coat the face and the normal pH balance is restored. Normal washing, no more than twice a day, cannot hurt the skin; overwashing, like most forms of overdoing, can.

Asking which soap is best is like asking which lipstick is best. It depends on who you are, on the condition of your own skin, and on what you want the product to do for you. A soap can be more than a cleanser—it can deodorize, perfume, or abrade your skin. I have several soaps—I use them for different parts of my body (except for my face)—and switch them with the season.

Mild or gentle soap. This refers to a soap that rinses quickly and easily from the skin after washing. Soap irritation results more from residue on the skin than from chemicals in the cleansing product. Any residue remaining on wet skin, even for a few moments, during the rinsing process is a source of irritation—and even of whitehead formation. Rapid rinsing, like fast lathering, is an important criterion for cleanser selection.

The Fast-Rinse Soap Test

A soap should rinse off quickly. A good test is often seen on television. Swish a bar of soap through a basin of water. Put your glasses, a mirror, or a plate in the soapy water. Then rinse quickly. Try this test with several soaps and you can easily tell which rinses off most quickly.

Here are some mild soaps I often recommend:

• Dove (Lever Brothers)
• Purpose (Ortho Pharmaceutical)
• Basis Sensitive Skin Soap (Beiersdorf)

Deodorant (antibacterial) soaps. These should be used only on the body, never on the face. Deodorizers kill the bacteria that normally feed on the perspiration of the apocrine sweat glands (for more on perspiration see chapter 24); since there are no apocrine glands on the face, there is no need to use deodorant soap on it. Deodorant soaps may also contain photosensitizing chemicals that can make skin vulnerable to sunlight. (For more about photosensitizing chemicals see chapter 6.)

Some soaps that prevent bacteria buildup:

• Hibiclens Antimicrobial Skin Cleanser (Stuart)
• Dial (Armour)
• Safeguard (Procter & Gamble)

Superfatted soaps. These have a high proportion of added fats that make a soap less alkaline, and so less disruptive to the skin's natural acidic film. Superfatted soaps are intended primarily for women with normal or slightly dry skin. If you have oily skin, superfatted soaps only make washing slower (they are oily so don't rinse quickly) and are less effective cleansers.

Two superfatted soaps:

• Oilatum (Stiefel)
• Eucerin (Beiersdorf)

Castile soap uses olive oil as a main fat; coconut oil soap uses coconut oil as its main fat. It is the *amount* of oil or fat used in a soap that makes it "superfatted"; some olive oil soaps are superfatted, some are not.

One castile soap is Maja (Myrurgia).

Transparent soaps. These are made with the addition of glycerine and alcohol and are widely promoted both for dry and oily skin. Both glycerine and alcohol, however, have the unique ability to draw water from the surface of the skin and dehydrate skin, making it tight and flaky after washing. These soaps are best for oily skin or the portions of the body that are oily.

The best known of the transparent soaps is Neutrogena (Neutrogena).

French-milled soaps. These are harder and more dense than other soaps. They often have a lower content of alkali as well. Milling is a process in which the soap is pressed when still soft to squeeze excess water and air from the bar. French-milled soaps go through two or three pressings, which concentrates the ingredients. Milled soaps seldom float, because they contain little air. Ivory (Procter & Gamble) floats easily; it is an airy example of an unmilled soap. The advantage of milled soaps is that they are long-lasting and lather extremely well. One example: English Lavender (Caswell-Massey).

Many of the so-called cosmetic bars that are part of a total skin-care program are French-milled. They are expensive, but last a long time. One example is Clinique's Facial Soap.

Synthetic soaps contain fatty acids that are derivates of petroleum chemicals instead of natural sources. This difference in composition doesn't affect their cleaning power, and because they are usually low in alkali they deposit less residue on the skin and rinse away very easily. They are usually kind to sensitive skin.

Soap substitutes are excellent for very sensitive skin. Included among them are:

- Lowila Cake (Westwood)
- Aveenobar (Cooper)
- Dove (Lever Brothers)
- Emulave (Cooper)

Exotic soaps. A wide variety of particles, grains, extracts, and perfumes are added to soaps. These ingredients are not all beneficial or harmless. Fruit, herbal, and perfumed soaps introduce potential irritants that you can well do without. A good rule is to avoid soap that is shaped like anything but a bar of soap or that smells like anything else, especially if you tend to have allergic reactions.

Non-Soap Cleansers

Detergents. It's very difficult to tell if you are using a detergent, a soap, or a combination. Detergents are often no harsher than soaps. Many rinse away quickly and completely and are excellent degreasers. The words *lauryl sulfate* in the ingredients indicate a detergent—if they are near the top of the list. If lauryl sulfate is included near the bottom of the ingredients list, the product is basically a soap.

Liquids are usually either detergents or less concentrated soaps. A liquid soap is at the other end of the hardness spectrum from a milled soap. Milky cleansers and washing creams and lotions are quite similar to liquid soaps; some simply have more water or oils in them, making them more liquid. Some products include camphor or menthol to speed evaporation and thereby make the skin feel cool and fresh. Unfortunately, this rapid evaporation depletes the skin's surface moisture and can lead to problems of dryness.

Grains added to soaps are given many names, but if the effect of the tiny particles within the cleanser is to whisk away dead skin cells, they are *scrubs*. In theory, scrubs are ideal for unplugging pores that are clogged with oil, old cells, or other debris, but the act of rubbing the surface of the skin may inspire the oil glands to produce even more oil and trigger acne in those who are susceptible, as well as damage the epidermis. Scrubs should be used very gently. At the slightest sign of irritation, stop.

Cleansers and Cleansing Creams

The line between liquid soaps and cleansing creams is very fine. Most cleansing creams contain a great deal of soap or an alkaline and oil combination of some kind, or they wouldn't clean the skin at all. Many cleansers are designed to be wiped away rather than washed away. Cleaning wipes may be useful in special situations but don't work well as a regular cleanser. The tissues leave some residue, which irritates the skin, and the wiping motions may stretch and stress the skin. Not using water deprives the skin of the benefits of water as a replenisher of its surface moisture. Regardless of what the label says, always rinse with water as a final step of cleansing.

Cold creams, Norcliff Thayer's Albolene, and other liquefying cleansers are variations of the same theme. They are formulated to remain solid in a jar at room temperature and to liquefy on the face at about 90°F. Because they liquefy, they are especially effective in combining with the oils and pigment in makeup and floating that residue away. Because they contain little or no alcohol, most liquefying creams are less drying than other cleansing creams.

The Basics of Cleansing for Your Skin Type

Oily skin—usually thick and shiny with large pores	Wash three times a day instead of twice. Never use so-called gentle or rich cleansers; they can bring on pimples. You can use hotter water, unlike people with other skin types. Use an astringent with a high alcohol content after each washing. Exfoliate twice a week.
"Normal" skin—moist, smooth, nonshiny; pores are hardly noticeable	No more than two washings a day. Use gentle cleansers. Avoid very hot water. Use a low-alcohol astringent or an alcohol-free toner after each washing.
Combination skin—oily T-zone, but normal or dry in other areas	Same care as "normal" skin. Use astringent on oily T-zone (nose, chin, and forehead).
Dry skin—usually thin; always feels tight after washing	Wash less frequently. Use a gentle or moisturizing cleanser and only luke-warm water. Watch out for acne-inducing cosmetics (see chapter 5).
Sensitive skin—thin; becomes red and irritated easily; may be sun-damaged; has a tendency to broken capillaries	Limit washings to once a day. Use a very gentle cleanser (like Cetaphil Lotion from Owen) and lukewarm water. Do not use abrasives such as washcloths, Buf-Pufs, grains; never rub dry with a towel. Never use toners or astringents with alcohol.

Presoaping Makes a Difference

Before you begin, secure your hair to avoid wetting it and getting makeup or cleanser into your hairline.

Start washing by using either a light oil (baby oil, some other mineral oil, or a commercial makeup remover) to loosen eye makeup, lip makeup, and other oily substances, so that your regular soap or skin cleanser can work more effectively. This preliminary step allows you to use less powerful and therefore less irritating soaps or cleansers.

Use your favorite cleanser and follow these steps:

- Wet your skin completely. Don't apply cleanser directly to your skin, but lather your hands and use your fingertips. (Brushes, washcloths, and loofahs are less clean than your freshly washed fingers—and less gentle.)
- Lather quickly, gliding the cleaning agent across the skin's surface. Don't scrub it into your skin. You want to dislodge old makeup, not force it farther into the skin. Wash quickly; don't spend more than a few moments.
- Rinse, rinse, rinse. Never reuse water from the sink basin—it is loaded with alkali and residue. Start your rinse with warm running water and gradually cool the water until it is as cold as can be tolerated. This tightens the surface of the skin and can make a strong toner unnecessary.
- Allow your face to partially air-dry before applying moisturizer. If the drippy feeling is unpleasant, pat dry with a clean white towel, avoiding any rubbing motion. Wet skin—like wet hair—is very elastic; it stretches easily and should be handled gently.
- Before moisturizing use a mild freshener, a toner, or an astringent—depending on your skin type—to make pores appear smaller and tighter. Apply the freshener, toner, or astringent with a water-soaked cotton pad to dilute the product's alcohol. Never use astringent in the eye or throat areas.
- Cleanse completely as many times as recommended for your skin type (see chart above). Be gentle—stroke softly and touch lightly. Lavish love on your skin; it will respond by looking great.

Cleaning Your Pores

For deep cleaning, try steaming your pores once a month. The easy steps:

1. Wash your face. Cleansing softens the contents of the pores and hydrates the skin.
2. Heat a teapot of water to boiling and let cool until the boiling stops.

3. Tent a towel over your head and stand with your face in the vapor from the spout at about ten to twelve inches away for five minutes.

Caution: Women with broken capillaries or a tendency to them should not steam their faces.

Cleansing Oily or Dry Skin

If you have oily skin, avoid cold cream and some much-advertised oily deep-skin cleansers. A gentle soap used consistently, with the occasional use of washing grains or other exfoliating cleansers, is probably what you need. Here are some products that may work for you (use only on chest or back):

- Acne-Aid (Stiefel)—a sulfated soap
- Acnaveen Cake (Cooper)—oatmeal, sulfur, and salicylic acid in a soap-free base
- Fostex Cleansing Bar (Westwood)—contains sulfur and salicylic acid

Picking or squeezing blemishes can lead to scarring. Just-washed moist skin can be damaged very easily; be careful.

If your skin is dry, choose superfatted soap for your body and a gentle cleanser for your face, and use less soap and more water.

Develop a washing routine that is right for you and your face will be forever grateful. Most of my patients overuse soap and underuse water. Make your soaps last a long time by using only a small amount. It is all you need.

4

WHY STRESS MAKES
MORE BUMPS THAN
WRINKLES

Does anxiety cause acne? It can and it does. I can almost read the amount of stress in the personal or professional lives of some of my patients by looking at their skin. Countless times I've seen a female patient who has suddenly developed a large blemish just before some important event. (It's happened to me too.)

The Hormone-Acne Connection

Hormones, those wonderful, mysterious chemicals that make you what and who you are, are manufactured in your endocrine glands. Many of the hormones that affect your skin come from your adrenal glands, which become more active when you are under stress and anxiety. When your adrenals are stimulated, they produce more male hormones. An excess of male hormones (the amount that is excess varies from woman to woman) can lead to acne. The adrenal glands do not distinguish between physical fear, stress, ordinary anxiety, or even great happiness, so almost any excitement can lead to blemishes. Type A behavior plays havoc with every body system, and the skin is no exception.

Both men and women produce male androgens and female estrogens. The sexes differ in the ratio of these hormones to each other. When the male and female hormone ratio in your body changes, as it does during growth spurts in your teens or other stressful periods, one of the results can be acne. Like many other women, you may recognize this phenomenon in your own skin. A few days before your menstrual period, when estrogen production is suddenly reduced, progesterone, which chemically resembles androgen, becomes more dominant and those premenstrual bumps appear.

Ovulation, menstruation, and childbirth sometimes stimulate acne formation, since the body often contains a higher androgen-to-estrogen ratio during those times. Certain androgen-dominant birth control pills such as Ovral and Lo/Ovral have a similar effect on the body.

Some women develop acne a few months after taking birth control pills; others notice flare-ups after abandoning that method of contraception. If you are in the first group, the synthetic progesterone (a hormone that behaves similarly to a male hormone) in your pill is probably the cause or a factor. The best solution is to switch pills to a different formulation. If you are in the second group, cheer up—your suffering is temporary.

Life-Style Acnes

Besides hormone changes, acne is encouraged or induced by dozens of natural activities or life-style patterns, habits, and events. Here are just a few.

Acne mechanica. This type is caused "mechanically" by rubbing, pressing, or irritating the skin with any material, including your own hands— resting your chin on your palm, for example, can cause chin bumps. (If you had hair follicles and oil glands in your palm, your palm might suffer too.) Other common causes are sleeping on your side or against your hand and leaning against a telephone.

Iodide and bromine acne. Artichokes, spinach, and kelp sound healthful but if you have any tendency to acne, you might do better eating a brownie. These high-iodide foods, and others like seaweed and shellfish, may activate acne when eaten in any quantity. Some soft drinks that contain brominated vegetable oils can also aggravate acne.

Fluoride acne. Be careful when brushing your teeth. Suds of fluoridated toothpaste can irritate the corners of your mouth, encouraging inflamed spots of acne on the chin and near the lips. Slosh mouthwash inside your mouth; don't allow it to touch your skin. Fluorides counter tooth decay, but they irritate the skin and can start a breakout.

Contraceptive acne. The new, safe, low-dose estrogen pills contain progesterone, a known sebum stimulator. Taking the pill—or quitting it—can cause hormonal changes. Either can trigger acne problems that may last for as long as two years—that's two years *after* you've quit the pill completely.

Medication and drug therapy acne. Through complex and different body mechanisms, the bromides and iodides in asthma relievers and cold pills, barbiturates, and tranquilizers all can affect the skin. Lithium, used in the treatment of some psychiatric disorders, may cause acne as well. Drugs used to treat epilepsy, tuberculosis, and some problems that involve hormone imbalances are known to be acne stimulators.

These are some of the drugs that can stimulate the development of acne:

Vitamin B_{12} Lithium
Phenobarbital (a sedative) Iodides
INH (an antituberculosis drug) Bromides
Phenytoin (used for the Danazol (a synthetic androgen
   treatment of epilepsy)   commonly used for the
Steroids   treatment of endometriosis)

Gourmet acne. Sautéing in butter, stir-frying in a hot wok, or just broiling over an outdoor grill exposes the skin to hot flying droplets of grease. The heat of cooking also stimulates your oil glands. Make your next outdoor barbecue a cold picnic. Steam your vegetables, and go easy on the butter.

Caribbean acne. Europeans call this Mallorca acne, after the Spanish island famous for its sunbathing tourists. Suntan and sunscreen oils applied to the skin may exacerbate acne (women seem to be more sensitive than men). The sun itself, though it dries the surface of the skin and evens skin color, often stimulates sebum production. Eight to ten weeks after your vacation, when your tan has already faded, the first tiny pustules of vacation acne appear, usually on the back and shoulders.

Clothing acne. Your favorite turtleneck sweater can give you acne. Wool and some synthetic fabrics irritate many skins—a combination of the friction of a heavy garment rubbing against your neck and back and your body's perspiration.

Steroid acne. Long-term steroid therapy, commonly used by athletes, can cause acne. A program that includes taking high doses of steroids by injection, orally, or even in the application of potent steroid creams to the face or body for a long period of time can result in acne.

Vitamin acne. This strikes the health enthusiast who lives on high dosages of vitamins, especially vitamin B_{12} injections or vitamin E taken orally. Multivitamins with minerals, particularly iodides, which are usually taken by pregnant women, may provoke acne. The acne will clear when the vitamins are discontinued. On the other hand, a vitamin B_2 or B_6 *deficiency* may also increase your skin's surface oiliness.

Food acne. Many commercially grown food animals are fed steroids that are chemically similar to androgens. When you eat large quantities of these foods your oil glands may be triggered and a side effect is acne. Wheat germ, peanuts, liver, kidney and other organ meats, gluten bread, and sweetbreads are foods sometimes associated with acne. Pork and lamb are usually safer than beef.

Makeup acne. The oils and other comedogenic ingredients in cleansers, makeups (concealers, foundations, or blushers), sunscreens, skin moisturizers (including lip moisturizers), and even unrinsed soaps can start the problem.

Fast-track acne. When the drive for success keeps you constantly impatient and chronically tense, you can get a case of acne along with your promotion. Stress can suppress estrogens, thus changing hormone balance. (An acnelike problem, acne rosacea, discussed in chapter 5, is another fast-track skin condition.)

Acne des jeunes filles. Hands off! Constant picking at tiny (or nonexistent) blemishes creates real blemishes.

Scrubbing acne. Frequent vigorous use of washing grains, brushes, and cloths stimulates the oil glands; scrubbing in an effort to free skin of excess oil can have just the opposite effect.

Hairline acne. Skin and scalp oils, conditioners, pomades, sprays, and other coatings, as well as cosmetics that are inadequately washed away from your hairline can cause a rash of whiteheads on the forehead. Apply conditioners only to the ends of your hair, since that is where they are most needed and where they have the least chance of contact with your skin. Bangs, side waves, and other on-the-face styles can bring on blemishes, too.

Headband acne is common among athletes who wear headbands across the forehead (leather bands are the worst because they don't allow skin to breathe); *backpack acne* can develop from the irritation of shoulder straps on the oily areas of the back and shoulders. Any outbreak of acne should inspire detective work. What could the culprit be? Which of your habits are making your pores clog? Which could cause the backup of oil and skin cells? Changing your habits can change your skin.

Nine Steps to Acne

Acne typically develops through a series of skin events:

1. If you are no longer a teenager, it may start with a change of some kind—perhaps a surprise or a disappointment.
2. Then comes a change inside the body's complex hormone system, which leads to a change in the balance of male to female sex hormones.
3. The male hormone level increases and stimulates the oil glands located within the hair follicles to enlarge and produce more oil.
4. Your face and hair become oilier; there is excess oiliness on the surface of the skin, especially in the T-zone.
5. Acne bacteria inside the follicles multiply and produce fatty acids, which irritate the lining of the pores.
6. There is also an increased number of thicker cells in the lining of the pores, and these tend to clump together.
7. This thickening narrows the pore openings, resulting in a backup of oil, skin cells, and debris inside the pores.

8. The pores clog.
9. The pressure from the clogged pores, constant production of oil, and irritation from bacterial action cause a rupture of the pore walls, which creates a blemish.

The birth of a blemish can take several days. The deeper the inflammation, the longer the pimple will last and the more likely it is to scar (very deep pimples are called cysts).

Blackheads and Whiteheads—The Same Problem with Different Hats

Dozens of diverse situations can set up the conditions so often triggered by hormonal changes. For example, oily makeup that blocks pores can also cause the backup of oil and debris.

The first sign of clogged pores is a blackhead or whitehead. Both are basically the same problem: comedones—plugs of dried sebum, cells, debris, and bacteria in the follicles.

In blackheads (open comedones), the plug has forced open the hair follicle or pore. The black tip is not dirt but oxidized oil. Very tiny comedones, which sometimes cannot be seen but are more easily felt, are called whiteheads. A whitehead is a closed comedone—a clogged pore still below the skin surface. Unlike a blackhead, the trapped oil, debris, and bacteria cannot escape. Both blackheads and whiteheads are plugs in the hair follicles. Since there are so many hair follicles and oil glands on your face, shoulders, chest, and back, there are endless opportunities for comedones of either type.

Fighting Acne on the Skin's Surface

It is possible to rid the skin of excess oil. Remember, though, that oiliness by itself does not cause acne and is actually good for the skin, and excessive scrubbing will only irritate the skin. Wash completely, gently, and carefully with a mild cleanser such as Cetaphil Lotion (Owen), which is oil-free. For shoulders and back use soaps that contain both drying and peeling agents. The drying agents will help to diminish oiliness; the peeling agents will loosen the plugs in the clogged pores.

Some good soaps for drying and peeling:

- Fostex Medicated Cleansing Bar (Westwood)
- Acne-Aid Detergent Soap (Stiefel)
- Neutrogena Acne Soap (Neutrogena)

SalAc (GenDerm), a new medicated cleanser, contains 2 percent salicylic acid and can prevent the development of blackheads and whiteheads.

Peeling Away the Problem

Another acne trigger is the buildup of cellular debris in the pores. The solution is to get the dead cells to move out faster, and thereby avoid traffic jams inside the pores. Skin peelers can help.

Sulfur, salicylic acid, and resorcinol as well as dozens of other preparations have been used for decades as skin peelers. Some have unpleasant side effects. Sulfur has something of a rotten-egg smell, and other chemicals and compounds can make the skin scaly, pink, and sore after use. These chemicals also have a tendency to irritate and inspire allergic reactions, so you risk trading acne for contact dermatitis. Dark-complexioned women, watch out: You should avoid products with sulfur and resorcinol, since both can leave your skin discolored and blotchy.

One skin peeler good for superficial pimples is Clearasil Adult Care (Richardson-Vicks).

The scrubs, grains, rubs, brushes, and pads that peel skin mechanically—very much the way pumice stone rubs away the skin on a callus—should be avoided for two reasons: Rubbing stimulates the oil glands, defeating your purpose; and rubbing affects only the skin surface. The backup of cellular debris is below the surface, in the follicles, so rubbing the surface doesn't do much good.

Benzoyl Peroxide

Of all the products used on acne, benzoyl peroxide, an antibacterial product available in both over-the-counter and prescription preparations, has been the most successful. It acts by releasing oxygen to kill bacteria attracted by the oil buildup in the pores. At the same time it has a drying and peeling effect and loosens blackheads to unblock pores. The bad news is that it can make your skin tender and sore, especially if it is used incorrectly.

If you check the labels on over-the-counter preparations for acne, you'll see benzoyl peroxide listed frequently. The higher the percentage of benzoyl peroxide and the higher the alcohol content, the more drying the product will be. It's best to start with a low percentage (the three strengths are 2.5 percent, 5 percent, and 10 percent), monitor your skin's reaction, and move on to higher percentages as your tolerance increases.

The following is a group of products containing benzoyl peroxide in varying concentrations.

	Percentage of *Benzoyl Peroxide*
Clearasil (Richardson-Vicks), cream and lotion	10%
Oxy (Norcliff Thayer), lotions	5 and 10%
Fostex (Westwood), gels	5 and 10%

Vanoxide (Dermik), lotion	5%
Loroxide (Dermik), flesh-tinted lotion	5.5%
Topex (Vicks Toiletry Products), lotion	10%
Erace Acne Control Cover-Up (Max Factor), stick	5%
PHISO AC BP Cream (Winthrop Breon)	10%

Over-the-counter benzoyl peroxide preparations are usually quite effective for small, superficial pimples. The main difference with prescription treatments—such as Desquam-X (Westwood)—is that they have a gel base and so are often more effective than over-the-counter products with cream and lotion bases. Some newer prescription products are also less drying (Persa-Gel W from Ortho Pharmaceutical, PanOxyl AQ from Stiefel, and Benzac W from Owen, for example).

A good way to use benzoyl peroxide is in washing bars that work like soap and can be used several times daily. They encourage peeling and leave skin virtually bacteria-free. However, I would recommend these only for oily parts of the body, not for the face. Two soaps that include benzoyl peroxide are:

• PanOxyl Bar (Stiefel)	5% and 10%
• Oxy Wash (Norcliff Thayer)	10%

For mild acne a benzoyl peroxide preparation may be all that is needed to keep bump-free. But don't expect immediate results. Results always take longer than you expect or hope. The treatment usually requires a minimum of three weeks of daily use for any noticeable improvement. Consistency counts; try not to miss a day.

Fair, thin-skinned blondes and women with mature or very delicate skin often find their faces become very dry, pink, and scaly in response to benzoyl peroxide treatment. If you're in this group—this product may not be for you.

Whenever you use a product containing benzoyl peroxide:

- Follow the directions on the preparations you use—exactly. If in doubt, use less rather than more.
- Avoid sensitive areas such as your upper lip, the corners of your mouth, around your eyes, your neck, and your earlobes (a woman's earlobes are often very sensitive—more than a man's).
- Never apply the preparation to damp skin, since moisture intensifies irritation.
- Don't use it if you will be exposed to cold or wind for any length of time.

Vitamin A Acid

For decades doctors have known that an excess of vitamin A will speed keratinization, the maturing of new skin cells. But only in the last dozen years has vitamin A acid been compounded so it can be used on the skin's surface with any great success. (It is used both in acne treatment and to improve older skin—because cell growth means new cells, and new cells mean younger cells and fresher-looking skin.) Vitamin A acid, chemically known as retinoic acid, is useful in the treatment of acne because it unplugs pores and reduces the cells' tendency to clump.

When you use vitamin A in a gel, cream, or liquid, the entire life cycle of a skin cell is decreased from about twenty-eight days to fourteen days or less. Speeding cell renewal is a way to prevent the clumping and clogging of the cells in the pores. Vitamin A acid may be used alone or combined with benzoyl peroxide—they work together beautifully, as the vitamin A acid helps to spur new cell growth and the benzoyl peroxide keeps the upper layer peeled smooth and fresh. Sometimes vitamin A acid is combined with a topical antibiotic (see below) and sometimes with both benzoyl peroxide and an antibiotic.

There is a down side to the use of vitamin A acid, however. Sometimes during the first weeks of application, dormant acne cysts and whiteheads under the skin may erupt and be rushed to the surface, and you'll look much worse than before. This period is temporary. Try to keep at it—you'll soon look better. Allow about six to eight weeks before expecting to see positive results. (If you are going somewhere really special in the next few weeks, wait to start the treatment until you have a relatively clear calendar for the next few weeks.)

Here are some things to remember when using vitamin A acid:

- Never apply it to wet skin; wait at least thirty minutes after washing your face.
- Use it very sparingly and avoid sensitive areas such as around the eyes and mouth.
- Apply it less often in cold, dry weather.
- Stop using it completely at least three days before you plan to be exposed to the sun for any time.

Vitamin A acid thins the skin by reducing the number of epidermal layers. Thin skin is not as good a protection from the outside world, especially the rays of the sun, as is thick skin. Follow your doctor's advice, and be very wary of the sun when you're using vitamin A acid; you are dealing with a potent medication. (See chapter 8 for more about this amazing, potent, and sometimes irritating vitamin derivative that requires a prescription and must be used only under a dermatologist's care.)

Medicated Astringents

An antibiotic astringent is sometimes used in combination with vitamin A acid and benzoyl peroxide for a successful acne-fighting regimen. These topical antibiotics help to destroy bacteria and decrease oiliness without irritation. They can be switched, depending on your needs, to be more or less drying. They are available only by prescription.

The following are among the antibiotic astringents available:

- Cleocin T (Upjohn); contains clindamycin   50% alcohol
- ATS (Hoechst-Roussel) 2%; contains erythromycin   66% alcohol
- EryDerm (Abbott) 2%; contains erythromycin   77% alcohol
- Staticin (Westwood) 1.5%; contains erythromycin   55% alcohol

For patients with skin sensitive to the alcohol in astringents, I prescribe Aknemycin (erythromycin) ointment from Hermal.

One new topical medication, Erycette Pledgets (Ortho Pharmaceutical), comes in the form of disposable pads treated with erythromycin solution, which you wipe over your face to clean it and kill bacteria. Another, Benzamycin Gel (Dermik), is a combination of erythromycin and benzoyl peroxide. Both are available only through prescription.

Combination Treatments

For most of us, regimens that combine skin-peeling, bacteria-destroying, and comedolytic agents work best. One of the best combinations I've found so far is vitamin A acid, benzoyl peroxide, and a topical antibiotic (medicated astringent). The vitamin A acid enhances the antibacterial action by allowing the other two substances to penetrate deeper into the pores, and it makes the benzoyl peroxide work even faster. But again, don't expect immediate results and do expect in the first weeks to have some irritation and peeling and a few more pimples than before. Progress means perseverance. Have courage and stick to it. Just as you don't lose much weight in a week, you can't get in shape in a week, good skin takes time, too.

Fighting Acne from the Inside Out

Bacteria Fighters

Since oil accumulation attracts massive numbers of bacteria and the bacterias' enzymes in turn produce fatty acids that irritate the skin, causing inflammation, one of the ways of battling acne has been to fight—and kill—the bacteria. Antibiotics—those "knights in shining capsules"—to the rescue, but by prescription only.

Antibiotics effective in the treatment of acne actually cut down the oil production of the glands slightly and destroy or decrease bacteria present in the follicles. The most popular are:

- Tetracycline, which must be taken one hour before or two hours after eating. Tetracycline binds to calcium, so don't drink milk while taking it. It should not be taken by children under ten, pregnant women, and mothers who are breast-feeding (because it can stain a child's developing teeth).
- Minocycline, which works better and faster than tetracycline.
- Erythromycin, which is prescribed for patients who don't respond to or are allergic to tetracycline. It can also be used during pregnancy.

The effectiveness of each antibiotic differs from one individual to another. Reactions are possible when any drug is used, so the best use is one limited in terms of quantity and duration. Among the array of side effects that have been noted with the use of antibiotics are:

Diarrhea	Rashes (including those induced
Nausea	by sun exposure)
Dizziness	Loosening of fingernails (after
Candida (vaginal yeast infection)	sun exposure)

When you are taking antibiotics it also makes sense to watch the food you eat. Alcohol alters the effectiveness of tetracycline, for example. Because tetracycline can deplete your body of vitamin C, make sure to take supplements. Avoid vitamins containing calcium, magnesium, aluminum, and iron, as these decrease the effectiveness of both tetracycline and minocin. Tetracycline and minocin also reduce the effectiveness of oral contraceptives. Use extra protection for birth control while taking these antibiotics.

Be sure to tell your doctor about other medications you use, and note your own reactions. Drowsy? Cranky? Sniffles? Don't dismiss any of these symptoms. What happens to you means something and it could be important.

13-Cis-Retinoic Acid (Accutane)

Read this carefully, and then read it again.

For severe forms of cystic acne (happily, a rare problem for women) that don't respond to regular treatment, Accutane, a potent vitamin A derivative that can be taken orally, has been developed. This new form of retinoic acid is in pill form and has been proven effective in the treatment of a high percentage of patients with cystic acne. *Caution:* One of the problems that has haunted vitamin A use is the fact that it can be toxic—and in some cases, when taken in megadoses, even lethal.

Before you rush to your dermatologist for a prescription, you should be aware of some of the side effects that are already known—and realize that the complete picture isn't in yet. Some of the side effects we do know about are:

- Dryness and cracking of the lips. Use lip balms or Carmex.
- Dry, fragile skin that cracks, breaks, and blisters easily at pressure sites. Heavy moisturizers are necessary, and 400 IU of vitamin E a day also helps diminish the dryness.
- Dryness of the mucous membranes. Eyes and nose are most affected; conjunctivitis, an inflammation of the eye, may occur. Use lubricating eye drops and petroleum jelly inside the nose.
- Increased susceptibility to sunburn. Sunscreens are a must.
- Joint pains, rashes, fatigue, migraine headaches, and elevated levels of fats in the blood. Dietary control is necessary (limit fats and alcohol; have blood levels checked monthly).
- Depression

But the major problem is a side effect affecting women only, Accutane's potential for causing birth defects. Accutane seems to have no effect on sperm.

When Accutane was first put on the market in September 1982, a clear warning appeared on the label and in patient brochures. The FDA had given Accutane an X rating—meaning it was a teratogen, an agent that causes birth defects. Dermatologists and pharmacists also received notices, but many young girls, not knowing they were pregnant or not wanting to tell anyone they were, took the drug. The warning says, "Do not become pregnant while using Accutane." *Take that warning seriously.* Pregnancy is not safe until two months after the course of medication is finished. There is even some concern about the reaction of nursing mothers to the drug.

Hormone Treatments

Regulating the androgen/estrogen balance may be a key to gaining some control of acne. Some women with oily skin and a long history of acne have been found to have an increased activity of the enzyme that converts testosterone, one of the male androgens, into a more potent form that affects the oil glands. A severe outbreak of acne, irregular menstrual periods, the growth of facial hair, personality changes, a dramatic weight gain, or a voice change should immediately be brought to the attention of a physician.

Anti-Androgen Therapy

Since androgens are implicated in the increased secretion of sebum that starts an acne blemish, doctors have tried to use drugs to counter the androgen action. Androgen blockers reduce the size of oil glands and cause hair to get finer and lighter and to grow more slowly in women with excessive hair growth. Anti-androgen therapy may be appropriate for women whose acne is associated with other changes such as hirsutism (excessive hair growth) or balding. (For more on anti-androgens see chapter 22.)

Steroid Injections

Intralesional steroids are extremely effective for inflammatory or cystic acne. A "disaster cyst" (my term for a large lesion that appears just before some public appearance or big date) can be stopped and healed in about twenty-four hours with a small amount of cortisone (usually Kenalog) injected directly into the lesion. The amount of cortisone needed and how it is injected can be judged only by an experienced dermatologist. The procedure is an art and a science, safe in the right hands, but not for experimentation. The injection is relatively painless, clears the skin rapidly, and prevents scarring.

Diet

Where acne appears to be provoked by foods (although genetic predisposition and other factors are usually in the picture as well), adjust your diet to avoid or limit known problem foods on your menu.

- Avoid high-androgen foods—beef, kidney, liver, sweetbreads, and other organ meats.
- Limit your intake of foods high in vitamin E—wheat germ bread, peanuts, and peanut butter are on that list. Shun salted nuts and crackers as party snacks; opt for raw vegetables and fruits.
- Avoid foods rich in halogen (a salt former, one of a group of compounds that also includes bromine, iodine, and fluorine, all with similar chemical properties). High-halogen foods include kelp, spinach, artichokes, and shellfish. Freshwater fish like brook trout are preferable to saltwater fish like tuna.
- Don't drink more than two glasses of milk daily and limit dairy products. (Cow's milk is high in progesterone.)

Remember the old wives' tale that greasy and fatty foods stimulate acne? That theory was discarded several years ago, but now it's making a comeback. Some women swear that chocolate or fries do make a difference; if you're among them, forget medical theory and stay away from your personal food enemies. (See chapter 17 for more details on diet.)

Other Acne Treatments

Sun Lamps—Don't Let the Sun Shine In

The use of ultraviolet lamps (instead of sun) used to be popular for the treatment of acne but is an outdated treatment. There are some obvious and hidden dangers you should take into consideration. Sun and phony sun in the form of fluorescent lights age skin and can lead to skin cancers. That's not all: There is real concern about the effect of ultraviolet lights on the eyes, since cataracts—the clouding of the lens—seem to be much more prevalent in sunny climates.

Surgery—Only When Done by a Professional

I use acne surgery routinely, usually starting on the second visit after the patient has used medications to unclog pores. Whiteheads especially require surgery, done with a comedone extractor, because they are under the skin's surface. The reason most cysts are opened is because there is less chance of scarring with surgery than with squeezing.

Don't be tempted to try "self-surgery" to unclog pores either by squeezing or with a commercially available extractor. I've never met a patient who has been able to do much more than further irritate an inflamed lesion by picking at it. And that's almost guaranteed to cause scarring.

Cold Treatments

Freezing the skin with liquid nitrogen or dry ice has been used as an acne treatment for dozens of years to produce exfoliation. The doctor uses powdered dry ice in a gauze bag (made by unfolding three handkerchief-sized gauze pads). The bag is first dipped in acetone and sulfur and then immediately applied to the skin with a sliding motion. It creates a temporary tiny and slightly painful frostbite where it touches the skin, and redness and peeling a few days later. Cotton swabs dipped in liquid nitrogen or sprays are also used. The treatment helps inflamed lesions dry faster but leaves comedones untouched.

Does it work? Yes, it works on any area with acne, but I find it works best on shoulders and backs.

Here's a good way to create coolness on your face without dried ice:

1. Fill your sink basin with cold water from the tap.
2. Put a trayful of crushed ice or cubes into a clean sock or wrap the ice in a towel. Weight the ice so it stays on the bottom of the sink.
3. Immerse your face in the icy water for as long as you can. A few good dunks of about thirty seconds at a time will help.

5

WHAT YOU CAN DO ABOUT ADULT ACNE

When you are too old to have it, too busy to fuss about it, and too anxious to take on even one more worry—adult acne strikes. And it is increasingly prevalent. Several years ago I might have seen a few cases of adult acne a year. Now I see dozens of cases in my office each month. At least half of all adult women suffer occasional breakouts. Triggered by stress and other modern phenomena, adult acne requires special attention. Besides the common acnes discussed in chapter 4, I'm also finding that women increasingly suffer from more "specialized" forms of skin blemishes.

Acne Rosacea

This acnelike condition, most prevalent in women and most severe in men, appears initially as a transient flush in the center of the face. The flush, whether fleeting or nearly permanent, eventually involves the cheeks and chin. The redness comes from the dilation of small blood vessels (vasodilation). Different from a blush because it is more intense and longer lasting, rosacea is rare in youth. The problem develops over a period of years.

Rosacea is often accompanied by oily skin, pimples, and sometimes dandruff. Because of the dilation of the blood vessels, small broken (permanently dilated) capillaries called telangiectasia, appear on the surface of the skin near the nostrils and on the cheeks. The redness may also affect the chin, but the shoulders and back are seldom involved. In severe cases rosacea can redden eyelids and the mucous membrane of the eyes, causing conjunctivitis. About half of all rosacea victims also suffer from burning and stinging eyes. Victims look flushed, blotchy, intense—and super emotional, which they often are.

What causes rosacea is not fully understood, but it appears to be aggravated by emotions. Genetic factors predispose some women to rosacea: Rosy, fair, and thin-skinned women with tempestuous natures are the prime candidates. Suppressing anger, fear, and other emotions adds to the number of flushes and increases the potential for eventual damage to the skin. Important occasions and ugly scenes can automatically trigger blushing and reddening.

Prevention Through Dietary Control

Rosacea-prone women are often wrongly suspected of drinking too much alcohol. It's much more likely that the high temperatures and spiciness of certain foods are at fault. Sipping cool water or icy drinks while you eat can help to avoid the flush. The temperature of the food is actually more detrimental than any spices in it—but a list of dietary no-nos is easy to compile.

Self-help should include a diet that restricts or minimizes spicy foods (they dilate the capillaries) and foods such as candy, pastry, and sugars, which are high in refined carbohydrates. (No one knows why these foods sometimes affect the skin, but they do.) The worst triggers for rosacea are those that contain histamine (a complex chemical found naturally in our bodies and in some plants and animals) or tyramine, both of which dilate the capillaries. Triggering foods and beverages include:

- Alcoholic drinks, especially red wine. Red wine, which contains histamine, is chemically different from white wine, which is okay. Beer, bourbon, gin, vodka, and champagne are also off your list.
- Sharp, aged cheeses containing tyramine, especially cheddar and camembert. Only cottage cheese is completely free of tyramine.
- Fermented, pickled, marinated, or smoked foods
- Chinese foods that are served very hot, have monosodium glutamate (MSG), or have soy sauce. (MSG may also be present in fast foods and some frozen foods.)
- Preserved meats with added nitrates, such as salami and a few other hard sausages. Bacon and hot dogs are also out because of sodium nitrate.
- Yeast extract
- Mustard, relish, raw onion, ketchup, sour cream
- Sour vegetables or fruits, especially citrus fruits, bananas, pineapples, figs, avocados, and tomatoes
- Raisins
- Peppers
- Vanilla extract
- Nuts

- Organ meats, especially liver
- Coffee, tea, and cola beverages

Nothing left to eat? Stick to bland, cool vegetables—turnips and cold potatoes are fine. Start with cold potatoes and gradually work your favorites back into your diet, monitoring your reactions as you go. When you have a reaction, strike the offending victual from your list. It's a bother and doesn't sound too appetizing, you say, but consider the consequences.

Life-Style Adjustments

Rosacea is stress- and emotion-related. Exercise dissipates stress, but it also raises the temperature of the skin and dilates the capillaries. Some good exercises for women with rosacea are bicycle riding, swimming in cool water, and even tap dancing. Find something you like that doesn't involve violent head movements or fierce competition. You don't need it.

The sun dilates blood vessels and aggravates rosacea, causing a flush and triggering small red papules. Keep calm, use sunscreens, and stay in the shade away from heat (both in temperature and emotion). Cool compresses similar to those used for sunburns (see chapter 6) can be applied at the first sign of flushing.

Self-Help

Here is my system for controlling rosacea, which you can modify for your own skin:

- Start by removing excess oil very gently, because your skin is already sensitive. Use a mild cleanser such as Cetaphil lotion (Owen), which is oil-free.
- Avoid washing in very hot or very cold water, so you don't either dilate or shrink the blood vessels—let them alone.
- Never use facial washing grains, brushes, washcloths, or abrading techniques.
- Steer clear of saunas, steam rooms, and hot tubs.
- Avoid exposure to the sun and always use sunscreens.
- Try to avoid becoming overheated.

After repeated dilations, blood vessels simply give up. They lose their ability to shrink to normal size and your face remains red. To tone down redness, a green-tinted light moisturizer or foundation can be used. The green neutralizes the red (if you mix green and red together you get beige). Ultima II (Revlon) and several other brands work well. Borghese's Velluto Liquid Toner goes on under makeup.

Sometimes masks are helpful because they absorb excess oil and include ingredients that soothe skin. Look for one or more of the following ingredients:

Allantoin	Ginseng	Rose hip
Calamine	Panthenol	Chamomile
Aloe vera	Azulene	Squalene

In severe cases medications can help. Rosacea responds well to antibiotics taken orally and other drugs such as Accutane. Here are some further suggestions:

- Avoid any cosmetics containing sorbic acid, which produces vasodilation.
- Avoid large doses of niacin, which stimulates the circulation of blood to the surface of the skin; try taking 10 milligrams of vitamin B_2 twice a day.
- When you take antibiotics (e.g. tetracycline, minocin, and erythromycin), you can expect the affected area to grow lighter and the oiliness to recede in about three to six weeks.
- Estrogen is sometimes prescribed for postmenopausal women who suffer from rosacea. Ask your physician about its use.
- A dermatologist can remove broken capillaries with a simple procedure.

To help conquer rosacea, relax! Take time to think of the big picture, don't let minor (or major) irritations ruin your skin. Have reasonable expectations of yourself and of others, and you'll find less to make you "see red" and be red.

Acne Cosmetica

Most of us are working women who use makeup to look good during days that start before 7 A.M. and don't stop—even for a minute—until midnight. (I sometimes have the feeling that if I sit down, I'll never have the energy to get up, so I keep going.) Yet many women find that cosmetics perform badly, causing acne cosmetica: The more you use makeup to look great, the worse it gets. Most vulnerable are women who suffered serious adolescent acne.

Cosmetics act several ways to set the stage for acne. However, it usually takes a few weeks to a few months after a culprit product is used to see lesions.

- Most cosmetics are somewhat occlusive—they seal the surface of the skin, denying passage in or out to air and moisture. Oil, unable to escape from a pore, backs up and clogs it.
- Almost all cosmetics contain some acne-stimulating oils or other substances that can cause certain individuals to develop blackheads and whiteheads (comedones).
- Cosmetics sometimes contain chemicals or colorants that irritate the skin and make it more vulnerable to acne.
- Inadequate cleansing leaves residue on the skin, which also can be irritating.

To avoid these problems, select your makeup carefully and apply it with techniques that avoid the side effects. Here is how to select and use cosmetics to minimize their acne-causing potential.

Moisturizer

Start by selecting a light, water-based moisturizer. Here are some to choose from:

- Keri Light (Westwood)
- Neutrogena Moisture (Neutrogena)
- Nutraderm (Owen)
- Shepard's Lotion (Dermik)
- Cetacort (Owen)

Sunscreen

If you use a sunscreen (and you should, even if your makeup includes its own sunscreen), check the label to be sure it is low in oils; the oils should be quite far down the list of ingredients. Vegetable oils, particularly olive oil, coconut oil, and cocoa butter, have a tendency to clog pores. Animal oils such as lanolin are often irritating as well as pore cloggers. Some noncomedogenic sunscreens are:

- Oil-Free Sunblock (Clinique)
- Total Eclipse Sunscreen Lotion (Herbert)
- Oil Free Tanning Gel (Elizabeth Arden)

Foundation

Any makeup foundation—cream, liquid, soufflé, or stick—can be troublesome if you apply it too thickly or don't wash it away carefully and completely.

Water-based foundations, unless oil-free, usually contain some oils, but less oil than oil-based products. The less oil in the makeup, the better it will be for your skin. To test your foundation for oiliness:

1. Apply a splotch about the size of a quarter to a sheet of 25 percent cotton (rag content) bond paper or to a plain brown paper bag.
2. Allow the makeup to dry thoroughly.
3. If no oily stain is left after the water in the makeup has evaporated, then the foundation is oil-free.

Water-based foundations don't provide as much coverage as oil-based products; those that require shaking to mix the pigments with the base are usually ideal for acne-prone women. These include:

- Natural Wonder Oil-Free Foundation (Revlon)
- BioClear (Helena Rubinstein)

- Pore Minimizer (Clinique)
- Pure Beauty Foundation for Oily Skin (Almay)

Also, look for the word *noncomedogenic* on the label.

I don't mind spending money on foundations. If you get the right one, it's the best investment you can make for you skin and your total look. To me my wardrobe of foundations—some oily for the outer edges of my skin on dry days, and some oil-free for my nose and forehead—is very important.

Acne Makeup

Applying makeup to disguise an acne flare-up will not exacerbate the problem or delay healing—*if* you use a medicated, skin-tinted acne makeup. Otherwise, you can expect trouble. Try these:

- Acnotex Lotion (C&M)
- Fostex Medicated Cover-Up (Westwood)
- Liquimat Lotion (Owen)
- Clearasil Regular Tinted Cream and Stick (Richardson-Vicks)
- Anti Acne Control Formula (Clinique)

Look for makeup that contains a high percentage of water, glycerine, or alcohol. (These ingredients should be near the top of the ingredient list.)

Don't be gulled into relying on such terms as *dermatologist-tested* (fine, a doctor was involved in the testing, but what were the results of the test?); *clinically tested* (the product was used in a clinic, but how many people used it, for how long, and, again, what was the outcome?); and *hypoallergenic* (the prefix *hypo* means "decreased," so *hypoallergenic* indicates that many known irritants have been removed, but not necessarily all of them).

Many high-priced and heavily advertised brands are loaded with acnegenic and comedogenic ingredients. The most exclusive gown looks odd if it fits poorly, and the same goes for cosmetics. Check your makeup labels. Although FDA regulations and good business practice have rid most cosmetics of common allergens and acne triggers, others remain.

Comedogenic Makeup Ingredients

These ingredients are to be avoided or used with caution by women with a tendency to acne. Some of these ingredients may be present in water-based cosmetics and even in acne medications.

Lanolin	Neopentanate	Octyl stearate
Decyl oleate	Myristyl myristate	Sodium lauryl sulfate
Isocetyl stearate	Isopropyl isostearate	Stearic acid
Isopropyl myristate	Myristyl lactate	Propylene glycol
Octyl palmitate	Butyl stearate	

Carry the list of comedogenic makeup ingredients to avoid with you when you are buying makeup. But remember it is often not just the presence of the ingredient but also its quantity in the product that is important. The lower on the ingredient list the less there is.

Eye shadows are seldom the culprits in acne cosmetica, because only a few modified oil glands are found in the eyelids. The cheeks and chin are the prime targets. Cream rouge is oilier than powdered rouge (blusher), because the pigments are held together with wax or oil. The cream can seep into pores and clog them, giving your skin a dotted surface. Select powder blusher unless you are always blemish-free.

Check the tiny labels on the backs of blusher packages. Read the small print. Avoid blushers with D&C (drug and cosmetic) red dyes. These are made from coal tar derivatives, potent comedone activators. Look for blushers made with iron oxide (Rubiglo is a popular brand). Carmine, a crimson pigment made from dried crushed Mexican beetles (yes, that's true), is also good.

Loose powders absorb oils more effectively than pressed powders. The best of the powders contain cornsilk, which blots up an amazing amount of facial oil without turning orangy as some other powders do. Apply your powder with a disposable cotton ball or a light brush that is washed often. (Wash your brushes in a few drops of baby shampoo, and dry them completely in a warm sunny spot.)

Perioral Dermatitis—Those Mysterious Spots Around the Mouth and Chin

If red, eraser-size bumps develop around your mouth you may be victim to a relatively new form of acne. Perioral dermatitis, first identified in the sixties, is becoming increasingly common among young women.

When you have this acnelike condition, the skin around your mouth is usually redder and drier than it is with ordinary acne. You may also have red bumps around your eyes.

Many experts believe that perioral dermatitis is in some way related to hormones secreted by the ovaries. Others note that the condition improves when fluoridated toothpaste is replaced with nonfluoridated. Still another theory links the condition with prolonged application of potent (fluorinated) steroid creams and greasy cosmetics. Women with a history of allergies and hay fever may be more prone to this condition and should avoid mentholated candy, cigarettes, lozenges, and chewing gum.

Perioral dermatitis requires treatment, as it generally does not clear up on its own, but there are steps you can take. Since drugstore over-the-counter acne fighters aggravate already dry and inflamed skin, stick to using a mild cleanser. Be careful not to touch or pick—your skin is supersensitive. Prescription antibiotics such as tetracycline, minocin, or erythromycin usually work. Here is a program that will gradually help:

- Thorough but gentle cleansing of the area is a must. If you use fluoride toothpaste, switch to a nonfluoride brand (Pepsodent, for example) and take care that not a smidgeon of foam touches your skin. Use a salt-and-water mouthwash that is free of fluorides. Also, be aware that some cities and towns pump fluoridated water.
- Avoid vitamins containing fluorides.
- Choose a water-based makeup. Don't wipe or rub your face with anything—especially facial tissues, which can lightly abrade your skin. Just blot.
- Use nongreasy moisturizers, for example Nutraderm (Owen) or Neutrogena Moisture (Neutrogena).
- In mild cases try over-the-counter preparations such as Lotio Alsulfa (Doak) and Fostril Lotion (Westwood). They can be used with cortisone creams or lotions such as Cortaid (Upjohn) or Dermolate (Schering).

In dealing with perioral dermatitis, adult acne itself, or any of the other acnelike problems, patience and forebearance are vital. Avoid extreme measures and rely on moderate ones. You're old enough to know that everything takes time.

6

KEEP YOUR SKIN
IN THE SHADE

I may leave home without my credit cards or even my house keys, but not without a sunscreen. I use a sunscreen every day, winter and summer.

The ancients believed in the magical properties of the sun. But the ancients didn't recognize the link between the sun and skin aging. The damage the sun can do depends on how many of the sun's ultraviolet (UV) rays actually reach your skin at any one time, and also on the cumulative effect of those rays. UV rays are shorter than visible light waves (which is why they are invisible) and they penetrate your skin only a fraction of an inch. But that tiny distance can make the difference between old and young skin.

The Burn Factors

Several factors regulate your skin's sensitivity to the sun.

Latitude. The closer you are to the equator, or the lower the latitude, the more direct and more concentrated the sun's rays are and so the more likely it is that you will get burned. When sunbathing in Minnesota, where the summer temperatures can reach to the 90s, there is less likelihood of being burned than sunning for the same amount of time in Puerto Rico, which is nearer the equator.

Time. The sun's rays are most potent at noon. Avoid exposure between 10 A.M. and 2 P.M. standard time; earlier and later hours of the day are less dangerous.

Temperature and humidity. Damage potential increases on a very hot day. If skin temperature is raised (during sports, for example) the sun's rays become more dangerous. On humid days when skin is moist and beads of perspiration stand on your nose or forehead, you burn more quickly.

Season of the year. More of the sun's rays reach the northern hemisphere at the end of June than at any other time of the year. Even warm days of the fall or winter are less dangerous than equally warm days in late spring or summer months. During winter months ultraviolet rays reach Earth at an angle that deflects some of the ability to penetrate skin.

Altitude. Thousands of feet above sea level the air is cleaner and thinner, with less protective atmosphere. The potential dosage of ultraviolet rays increases about 5 percent for each 1,000 feet above sea level. If you are exposed on a mountain top near the equator, ultraviolet rays can be disastrous, and mountain people are often victim to skin cancer.

Pollutants. Each tiny particle of dust, dirt, and debris in the atmosphere around us can absorb ultraviolet rays and protect skin from the effects of the sun. In a smoggy place the atmosphere provides protection from a high percentage of the ultraviolet rays.

Clouds. On a cloudy day, skin still can receive as much as 60 percent of the sun's ultraviolet rays.

Winds. High winds intensify the effects of the sun's rays.

Background surface. Any reflective surface can magnify the sun's rays: Water, cement, sand, or any smooth, shiny surface can encourage more damage than grassy, dark, or dull surfaces. Clean white snow reflects a large percentage of ultraviolet rays. Using a metallic mirrorlike reflector invites sun damage.

Water can be penetrated by the sun's rays. Only scuba divers who swim twenty feet or more beneath a murky surface can consider themselves safe. Outdoor pool swimming amplifies the sun damage factor.

Skin surface. Your own skin can form a barrier: Thick skin and dark skin offer more protection than thin and light skin. The V of your neck, your breasts, and shoulders are the most sun-sensitive areas, but the protruding areas—nose, ears, cheekbones—are very susceptible to burning. Your own skin is a natural barrier against ultraviolet rays—a suntan offers a sun protection factor (SPF) of about 3—but it still needs all the help you can give it and all sun exposure is potentially damaging. Whenever I see a woman of any age sunning I can hardly control the urge to rush up and shout, "Stop! Don't you know you are damaging yourself?"

Age. Usually, after forty you grow less vulnerable to sunburn.

Activity. Whether you're active or not also makes a difference. If you're upright and moving around, you'll get less ultraviolet light than if you're lying down sunbathing.

Fabric. The fabric your clothing is made of can make a great difference in how much protection you receive against ultraviolet rays. The more tightly woven a fabric, the more protection it offers. Cotton, for example, with its tight weave offers much more protection than the loose weave of synthetic materials.

A word of caution about the Unsuit Bathing Suit: This suit is constructed to allow the sun's rays to penetrate, but though the manufacturer has assigned a sun protection factor of 6 to the suit, dermatologists consider it closer to 3. It is wise to wear a sunscreen under the suit as well as on exposed skin to avoid "unsuited sunburn."

Oil or water (or a moisturizer) can encourage sunburn. Shiny surfaces act as a lens, magnifying rays. Applying an oily moisturizer without a sunscreen can invite more damage than wearing nothing at all.

Medicines and foods. Some foods and drugs can affect your skin's sensitivity to ultraviolet rays. There are two types of sensitive reactions to the sun that can be triggered by food or medicine.

- A phototoxic response affects the victim at once. As soon as you go in the sun a red puffy reaction similar to a bad sunburn appears, but there is no itch or burning sensation.
- A photoallergic reaction requires a few exposures to the sun. It looks more like eczema or poison ivy, and always itches—sometimes terribly. Fortunately, this kind of reaction is quite rare.

The list of products that have the potential for photosensitizing the skin grows every day. The following chart lists only some of the known sensitizers. It is far from complete; photosensitive reactions to foods, drugs, and dyes are discovered daily.

Sun-Reacting Agents
Medicines

Type of Drug	Includes
Antibacterials	Deodorant soaps, some germicides (containing halogenated salicylanilides)
Antibiotics	Doxycycline, tetracycline, minocycline, oxytetracycline, chlortetracycline or any derivatives
Anticonvulsives	Carbamazepine, trimethadione
Antidepressants	Amitriptyline, desipramine, doxepin, nortriptyline, protriptyline
Antidiabetics	Sulfonylureas found in tolazamide, chlorpropamide, tolbutamide

Type of Drug	Includes
Antihistamines	Diphenhydramine, cyproheptadine. (If you plan a trip to the tropics you should be aware that some motion-sickness remedies can encourage sunburn.)
Antifungals	Griseofulvin
Bromides	Used in sleep aids
Cardiac agents	Quinidine
Nonsteroidal anti-inflammatory agents (used for menstrual discomfort and arthritis)	Piroxicam, sulindac, Naproxen
Diuretics	Furosemide, thiazides
Dyes	D&C red dyes (often found in lipsticks and blushes), eosin, fluorescein, methyl violet, methylene blue, orange-red, rose bengal, toluidine blue, trypan blue
Estrogens and progesterones (birth control pills or hormones)	Mestranol and norethynodrel, diethylstilbestrol
Perfumes and toilet waters	Oil of bergamot, oil of cedar, citron, lavender, lemon, lime, rosemary, cinnamon, and sandalwood
Antibacterial agents	Sulfanilamide, sulfacetamide, sulfadiazine
Sunscreening agents	Para-aminobenzoate and cinnamate (in rare cases, shown to be the cause of photocontact allergic dermatitis)
Tars (included in many psoriasis medications and some over-the-counter shampoos and bath products)	Coal tars, coal-tar derivatives, wood tars, and some petroleum products
Tranquilizers	Phenothiazines
Urinary antiseptic	Nalidixic acid

Foods

Furocoumarins are a group of chemical substances that are often highly phototoxic. They include surprising foods: parsnips, celery, carrots, figs, many different greens, cyclamates (banned in many calorie-free drinks but making a comeback due to new FDA studies), tonic drinks with quinine. (See chapter 11 for more about photosensitizing foods.) Artificial sweeteners such as saccharin may be responsible for photosensitive reactions because they contain sulfa.

The ABCs of Ultraviolet Rays

There are differences in ultraviolet light, and they affect the way your skin tans and ages.

Ultraviolet A (UVA) in large doses produces mild redness of the skin almost immediately, but its effects disappear within a day. This is the slow tanning ray: Although weaker than ultraviolet B in terms of its burning effect on the skin, it does age skin, penetrating deeper into the dermis than other rays. UVA rays are directly responsible for freckling, most phototoxic and photoallergic reactions, and premature skin aging. These silent rays penetrate glass, water, and plastic barriers, adding to skin aging. The A rays also intensify the damage potential of the B rays. Every time you step near a window, outdoors, or even under a fluorescent light, you're contributing to your total exposure to A rays.

Ultraviolet B (UVB) of the midday sun causes the severe burns. The signs of redness from ultraviolet B appear between three and eight hours after exposure and start to fade about twelve hours later. (That's just when your sunburn shows up, so it is easy to tell how severely your skin has been damaged.) If a very high dose is received, your skin can remain red for as long as a week, or even longer. UVB is the sunburn ray associated with liver spots and skin cancer.

Ultraviolet C (UVC) is the least penetrating. The color you get from it usually peaks at about eight hours after exposure and fades quickly. Only small amounts of C light reach the Earth, while about 10 to 20 percent of B affects the skin and about 50 percent of A enters the dermis. It is this penetration that causes accelerated aging.

Is there any excuse for sunbathing? If you're still not completely convinced, read on.

Some evidence supports the theory that ultraviolet light rays A and B and even C can adversely affect the skin's genetic material, deoxyribonucleic acid (DNA). UVB is considered most damaging of all. No tan—no matter how light, how even, and how carefully cultivated—is healthful.

What's Your Tan Type?

Your tan type can be almost as important as your Social Security number. For ease in classification, six basic reactions to the sun are used to describe how people tan. The types are consistent with eye color, hair color, and the melanin content of skin.

Type 1. You don't tan—you always burn. Your skin is very light and thin. You probably have blue, green, or hazel eyes; your hair may be blond or red. You freckle easily; your sunburn remains red for a long time. Always wear a sunblock or sunscreen with a sun protection factor (SPF) of 15 for the face and exposed parts of the body.

Type 2. Your skin is fair and you might have blond or light brown hair and blue, gray, or hazel eyes, but you do tan a little—if you approach it very gradually. Always wear SPF 15, at least on the face.

Type 3. You have blond to brown or black hair and medium to fairly dark skin. Although you are slightly sensitive to the sun, you tan well and can enjoy the sun if you use a sunscreen. You may be what is called a California blonde. You're very vulnerable in early spring or on a midwinter vacation. Wear a sunscreen with SPF 15 on the face, SPF 10 on other areas.

Type 4. You are probably a brunette with olive skin tones. You tan easily; you've never had a bad burn. Don't be overconfident; your skin still can be damaged by the sun. You should choose an SPF of 8 to 10.

Type 5. Gold-toned or beige skin can take large quantities of sun before the UVB causes burning; but you can burn, and your complexion can also be damaged by brown spots and other solar marks. Use an SPF of 6 to 8.

Type 6. Dark brown or black skin means that you almost never burn. However, an application of sunscreen—SPF 2 to 4—will keep your skin younger-looking longer.

No matter what your tan type, you should be fully aware that you're courting aging skin every time you venture unprotected into the sun. T-shirts, light clothing, and especially loosely woven clothing offer almost no protection from burning rays. Keeping sun exposure hours to early morning and late afternoon helps somewhat. (Don't get too confident—the slower UVA tan can still leave your skin sagging and damaged.)

Recently when examining a new patient, I asked, "When did you suffer that severe sunburn?" She was amazed that I knew in fact that she had been burned fifteen years earlier. She hadn't realized that the effects were visible on her skin in the form of giant so-called sunburn freckles, usually found on the shoulders, chest, and back.

The cumulative effect of sun damage is well documented. Although it doesn't show up until later in life, it starts in your teens. Youthful burns may only damage a small percent of your skin cells, but the count goes on through your entire life—adding to that destruction.

Sunscreens—Help When You Need It

Sunscreen products were first introduced over forty years ago. They're ultraviolet ray absorbers that use para-aminobenzoate (PABA), and have been tested over the years and are usually safe and effective. Since then, hundreds of products have been introduced. Sunscreens work in several ways: Some, called sunblocks, reflect the ultraviolet rays by providing a shield on the surface of the skin; others, sunscreens, absorb the harmful rays by creating a chemical barrier.

An ideal sunscreen should:

• Be invisible to ordinary view; inpenetrable to ultraviolet light
• Adhere, allowing you to swim and engage in sports in the sun
• Not stain clothing
• Remain stable and not change chemically once applied
• Not cause irritation or allergic reaction
• Be odorless, nongreasy, nondrying, and inexpensive

A "sunscreen pill" is in development, because experiments with animals show that it is possible to block rays and minimize sunburn reaction, as well as its effects, with an oral sunscreen. But until a pill is perfected, sunscreens should be used by everyone—with complexions from alabaster to ebony. A sunscreen cannot be *too* protective.

SPF (Sun Protection Factor)

The effectiveness of all sunscreens is announced by labels describing the product's SPF (sun protection factor) and generally using the numbers 2 through 15 (numbers higher than 15 don't offer significantly more protection). To arrive at SPF the manufacturers run indoor tests on people with the six basic skin types. The number indicates how much time you can safely spend in the sun without fear of burning if you have applied the product. For example, if a product has an SPF of 2, you can spend twice the amount of time in the sun without getting burned as you could without an application.

If you are Type 4 and don't burn easily, you might normally be able to spend twenty minutes in the sun without reaction; with an SPF 2 product you can spend twice that time, or 40 minutes:

20 minutes × SPF number (2) = time in the sun without burning (40 minutes)
$$20 \times 2 = 40$$

The lower the SPF number, the more rays reach your skin. Remember you will still tan with an SPF of 15. For better protection it is advisable to use a sunscreen with a higher SPF number than you think you need. See the box on page 57 for sunscreens that protect against both UVA and UVB rays.

Sunblocks are barriers that scatter (reflect and bounce the light, just as a tennis ball bounces against a hard surface) all the light in the ultraviolet range. When the rays are scattered, sunburn is prevented or minimized. Abnormally sensitive reactions to all light are lessened. The zinc oxide that lifeguards use on lips and noses is an example of a sunblock.

How to Use a Sunscreen

The degree of protection from any product, whether its SPF is 2 or 15, also depends on how you use it, how often you apply it after swimming or sweating, how humid the environment is, and the other various factors listed at the beginning of this chapter.

You can even buy a sun-exposure meter (the Ultraviolet Sensor from Teledyne), which adjusts to your skin type and measures the sun's rays, signaling when your time in the sun is up.

To get the best protection from your sunscreen, follow these guidelines:

- If you use the product on your face, apply it over your moisturizer but under your makeup. (In that way your skin will be protected by your moisturizer, but the cosmetic surface texture of your foundation will not be affected.) If the sunscreen has a moisturizing base, skip your moisturizer.
- Don't rub any sun product into your skin; stroke it on with a one-directional movement. (The barrier of a sunscreen should be over your skin's surface, not rubbed into your skin's pores.)
- Apply all sunscreen products at least an hour before exposure; since the products have a cumulative effect, it is wise to apply sunscreens daily to exposed parts of your body. Reapply every two hours, more often if you exercise or swim. (You're always exposed to some kind of ultraviolet light—it might be smart to make a sunscreen part of your daily grooming.) Not applying it generously lowers a sunscreen's SPF.
- Watch for adverse reactions: Just as with other cosmetic products, experiment to find which is best for you.
- Regular application is a must.

Matching Your Sunscreen to Your Skin

Most sunscreen chemicals are not soluble in water, so an alcohol base is used. If your skin is very dry or sensitive, alcohol in the product will dry your skin even more. Newer formulas often use an oil base, which better adheres to the skin—especially a swimmer's skin. Acne-prone women should use alcohol-based sunscreens because the heat of the sun combined with the oily base can aggravate your skin more than help it. Sunscreens containing PABA can stain clothing—yellow spots occur where the clothes are exposed to the sun; linen and cotton fabrics stain most easily. Sunscreen with PABA esters rather than PABA will not stain clothing.*

Matching a Sunscreen to Your Skin Type

Skin Type	Sunscreen
Oily skin: Use alcohol-based lotions or gels.	Presun 15 (Westwood) Pabanol (Elder) Sea & Ski Block Out (Carter) Pabafilm (Owen) Total Eclipse Sunscreen Lotion SPF (Herbert)
Dry skin: Use creams or moisturizing lotions; avoid alcohol-based products.	Piz Buin 8 (Greiter) Bain de Soleil (Charles of the Ritz) Total Eclipse Moisturizing Lotion (Herbert) Suncare Sun Blocking Cream (Elizabeth Arden) Nivea Moisturizing Sun Block Lotion (Beiersdorf) Presun Facial Sunscreen (Westwood)
Combination skin: Use alcohol lotions for oily T-zone and creamy lotions for normal and dry areas.	
Acne-prone skin: Avoid sunscreens that contain cocoa butter or coconut oil.	Oil-Free Sunblock (Clinique) Oil-Free Tanning Gel (Elizabeth Arden) Oil-Free Tanning Formula (Estée Lauder) Oil-Free Ultra Block SPF 15 (Elizabeth Arden)

*For further information about protecting your skin from the sun, the American Academy of Dermatology at 820 Davis Street, Evanston, IL 60201, has an excellent free pamphlet titled *The Sun and Your Skin*.

A Mini-Guide to Some Sun Preparations

These products minimize tanning and prevent burning (UVB protection only):
- Pabafilm (Owen)
- Sundown 8 (Johnson & Johnson)
- Sea & Ski Block Out (Carter)

These products prevent phototoxic reactions (UVA protection only):
- Uval (Dorsey)
- Solbar (Person & Covey)

These products prevent sunburn and sun-related aging (both UVB and UVA protection):
- SunGard (Dome)
- Presun 15 (Westwood)
- Sundown 15 (Johnson & Johnson)
- Supershade 15 (Plough)
- Clinique 19 (Clinique)
- Total Eclipse Sunscreen Lotion SPF 15 (Herbert)
- Bain de Soleil 15 (Charles of the Ritz)
- Suncare Sun Blocking Cream 15 (Elizabeth Arden)

These products provide the maximum protection for your skin. They are sunblocks (and are usually opaque):
- Zinc Oxide Ointment, USP (Pharmaderm)
- RVPaque (Elder)
- RVPlus (Elder)
- Sunblock Creme SPF 23 (Estée Lauder)
- Solar Cream (Doak)
- Continuous Coverage (Clinique)

Waterproof sunscreens:
- Sundown 8 and 15 (Johnson & Johnson)
- Supershade 15 (Plough)
- Clinique 19 (Clinique)
- Coppertone 15 (Plough)

Allergies and Sunscreens

Some women are allergic to PABA and its esters. If you are allergic to the "-caine" group of anesthetics (lidocaine, benzocaine, etc.) or to certain hair dyes (those containing paraphenylenediamine) or sulfonamides, you might be allergic to PABA. (Often the allergic reactions look like a sunburn, making the cause difficult to determine.) If you think you might be allergic to PABA, use a PABA-free sunscreen such as one of the following:

- TiScreen Lotions SPF 8 and SPF 15+ (T/I Pharmaceuticals)
- Solbar (Person & Covey)
- Uval (Dorsey)
- Piz Buin 8 or 15 (Greiter)

Vitamin E has recently been discovered to be an effective sunscreen ingredient. It reduces sun-induced damage, but it can trigger acne when applied topically.

There are more than twenty different chemicals that the FDA recognizes as safe, effective sunscreen ingredients; success depends on how well, how often, and how consistently any of them are used. Some of these are:

- PABA and PABA esters—UVB filters
- Cinnamates—also absorb UVB; can cause contact and photocontact dermatitis
- Salicylates (such as homomenthyl salicylate)—absorb UVB; may cause contact dermatitis
- Benzophenones (oxybenzone, sulisobenzone, mexenone)—absorb UVA
- Anthranilates (menthyl and homomenthyl-N-acetyl)—absorb UVA

Treating Sunburn

Ultraviolet rays penetrating unprotected skin can trigger electrochemical reactions that cause epidermal cell death. The acute effect of the sun on skin is sunburn, and any severe sunburn indicates damage to the epidermal cells and to the blood vessels that feed them.

Dehydration of surface skin cells is usually part of the discomfort of a sunburn. Sunburn can be a slight pink tenderness that vanishes the next day or a painful blistering that may take two or three weeks to remedy. You should treat sunburn with the same seriousness as you would any skin problem.

When overexposed to the sun, first evaluate the damage; then decide on the best course of action. Examine the skin and note its color.

Color	Problem	Help
Pink/redness usually appears 12 hours after exposure; local heat and burning	Mild sunburn (disappears within a day or two)	Soothing, cool compresses or soaks of equal parts of milk and water; ice cubes can be added; refrigerated moisturizer will soothe and relieve dryness.

Color	Problem	Help
Red, tender areas; outlines of clothes visible; itching and stinging	Moderate sunburn	Aspirin; moist compresses twice a day for 20 minutes of Burow's solution, made of Domeboro tablets or powder (available at drugstores); OTC steroid creams (such as Cortaid and Dermovate)
Red, swollen, glistening skin; painful blisters and oozing that continues for days; fever, chills, nausea	Severe sunburn (2nd-degree burn)	See a dermatologist! Moist compresses; cool baths with oatmeal; systemic corticosteroids (by mouth or injections)

If you even *suspect* a severe sunburn, find reliable medical help.

Home Relief for Sunburn Pain

For the first few hours after overexposure to the sun the redness and sensitivity can be relieved by applying a variety of preparations.

- Moisturizers to prevent further skin dehydration (refrigeration makes them more soothing)
- Skin preparations containing phenol, menthol, or camphor for cooling. Sarna Lotion (Stiefel) is one such preparation.

Drink lots of water to replace lost body fluids.

Cornstarch, sprinkled on sheets to minimize friction, will make sleeping more comfortable at night.

Compresses also provide relief. They can be made from handkerchiefs, pillowcases, or pads of gauze; the cloth should be lightweight and comfortable, even when wet. Wet the compresses by dipping in a liquid solution, then drape the cloth over the affected area. Allow the solution to evaporate. You can direct a fan on the sunburned area to heighten the cooling.

Some easy home care compress solutions:

- Lukewarm tap water can be used on unbroken skin.
- A cup of milk added to about a cup of lukewarm tap water increases the latter's calming effect.
- Salt water. Salt is a humectant (a substance that attracts and holds moisture). Add a half teaspoon of salt to a quart of tap water to make a compress solution.

- Oatmeal soothes the skin and stays moist a long time. Put a half cup of cooked oatmeal into a quart of lukewarm water. Soaking in a tepid bath into which oatmeal has been added is also soothing.

I've often advised patients to apply ice water, ice milk, or witch hazel compresses to the eyelids, lips, or other sun-vulnerable areas. Sometimes a suffering patient will call to tell me she or he got almost instant relief from just a moist, icy compress.

Slices of apple, raw potato, or cucumber are folk remedies that work for many. They are all slightly astringent and may reduce inflammation. Just slice the fruit or vegetable and pat your sunburned skin with the moist slice. Follow with a cooling rinse of water. Aloe vera gel from a cut aloe leaf may also soothe a sunburn.

Avoid using soap on burned areas. Also, don't use butter or other greasy substances or ointments, which may then be painful to remove.

If you are very uncomfortable and need a topical anesthetic, you can try Prax Lotion (Ferndale Labs), available without prescription.

Aspirin Can Reduce a Sunburn

Aspirin suppresses inflammation by opposing the formation of biologically active body substances called prostaglandins, which are linked with swelling, burning, and pain. Provided your physician allows it, two tablets of aspirin taken three times a day *prior to* sun exposure can suppress the heat and redness of sunburn. Don't try to substitute Tylenol or other aspirin substitutes. They don't work the same way. Indocin (indomethacin) (Merck Sharp & Dohme) is a prescription drug that also can reduce the potential severity of sunburn when taken before exposure.

Don't Take Sunburn Lightly

A severe sunburn is a major medical emergency and should not be treated casually. If you're away from home—and that is when these sunburns usually occur—call a member of the local medical group or the hotel physician. As a last resort you can go to the emergency room of a local hospital. If the burn is extensive, you may be hospitalized so that compresses, emollients, or antibiotics can be used to speed healing and avoid complications. Corticosteroids, indomethacin, or antihistamines are often prescribed. As with any burn, the initial healing may take weeks—and the damage to the skin may be irreparable.

Sun Poisoning

Sun poisoning is not a medical term but just the way many people refer to severe sunburn. Watch for these signs if you are burned:

- Shocklike state of dehydration caused by excessive evaporation of body fluids

- Dilation of the skin's blood vessels
- Raising of the surface temperature of the skin
- Increasing body temperature (a fever)

Temporary home relief until you can reach a physician usually includes:

- Drinking water and fruit juices
- Reducing pain and inflammation with aspirin
- Immersing the body in a tepid bath to which Aveeno Oilated Bath (Cooper) or Alpha Keri Therapeutic Shower and Bath Oil (Westwood) has been added. (Do not use soap; it will strip skin oils.)
- Rest

Nausea, faintness, and fever are not uncommon in severe sunburn. If there is persistent itching, take Chlor-Trimeton tablets (Schering). In the worst cases your doctor may prescribe a potent anti-inflammatory drug (steroid) such as prednisone, which should be taken by mouth for about three to five days.

Sunless Tans

Although dark tans are less popular than they once were, some women still want a tan—without the damage. Skin stains from natural products like tea, juglone from walnut juice, and lawson from henna have been used for hundreds of years, and modern artificial tanners are on the market in great numbers. DHA (dihydroxyacetone), used for over twenty years, produces a yellow-brown shade and cannot be washed away, although it does fade as the epidermal cells are sloughed off with the outer layers of the skin. It is found in Coppertone's QT (Schering Plough), Sea & Ski Indoor Tan (Carter), and Self Action Tanning Creme (Estée Lauder). French and German firms have produced skin tanners in a wide variety of skin colors, from brown to yellow gold. Very simple options for a fake tan are bronzing gels, which are just makeup color or tinted moisturizers applied to the skin.

The unsafe factor associated with artificial tanners is the feeling that it's safe to sunbathe because you're already tan, but it's actually not safe.

Tanning pills containing canthaxanthin, a dye that changes skin color, are also available. However, they carry a very stiff warning from the FDA that canthaxanthin is unsafe taken orally and can accumulate in the blood, skin, fatty tissue, and organs such as the liver.

Sunlamps can also produce a tan. They have about the same effect as midday at midlatitude in summer, as they are a source of mostly UVA light. While useful in the treatment of psoriasis, they can cause premature aging and chronic skin damage, including skin cancer, and so are questionable to use. The dangers of this kind of radiation cannot be ignored. One of the most obvious hazards is to the eyes (there is an increased risk of cataracts). If you use a sunlamp, always wear dark glasses (Noir chemical sunglasses offer good protection), and never look directly into the light.

Reversing the Damage

Can the damage of years past be reversed? The latest evidence suggests hope. A recent experiment contrasted biopsies of sun-caused tumors with biopsies done on the same people after several years of sun avoidance. Most of the tumors noted in earlier biopsies had regressed, and the structure of the skin had improved, indicating that with the absence of ultraviolet radiation the skin can reverse the cancer-developing progress. (This is not to suggest that any skin lesion should go unexamined by a dermatologist.) Thus, no matter how much of a "misspent youth" was enjoyed in the sun, it is possible to prevent further damage and to achieve some degree of improvement.

Retinoic acid (Retin A) in cream and gel form has recently been reported helpful in reversing sun damage because of its ability to speed up cell regrowth and possibly even repair collagen of sun-damaged skin to some degree.

Premalignant Lesions

Solar, or actinic, keratoses can appear on sun-exposed areas of the body. These sun-caused lesions are red, scaly, and rough to the touch. Initially flat, they can become raised and malignant in time (though they grow slowly and it make take decades for them to become malignant). An itching, thickened, or bleeding lesion should send you to your dermatologist as soon as possible.

Periodic self-screenings of your skin is a new concept but a valid one. I believe you need both a full-length and a hand-held mirror, a good light, and a friend or a mate (for hard-to-see places). Look for unusual moles, blemishes, sores, or discolorations. Among the warning signs of skin cancer are a skin growth that appears suddenly or increases in size.

Solar keratoses are either treated surgically or with 5-FU (5-fluorouracil) solution or cream. This agent seeks and destroys damaged cells, leaving normal ones alone. With this treatment the skin will at first become red, tender, and crusted (topical steroid creams can be used to soothe) and some previously invisible keratoses may be unmasked. But after a short period of discomfort, 5-FU should leave you with improved skin without scarring.

Skin Cancers

Close to half a million cases of skin cancer are reported every year—and many more go unreported. The incidence of skin cancer has doubled during the past twenty-five years, increasing at an alarming rate. At one time most cancers appeared on older people, but today I see many patients in their thirties who already have cancers of the skin.

It takes years for skin cancers to develop, because they result from cumulative exposure to ultraviolet light. For this reason I remind mothers to use sunscreen on their children whenever they go outdoors, from six months on.

Sunlight is the principal cause of skin cancer, but there are other less common causes: X rays, coal tars, and arsenic among others. Don't panic when you notice some small mark or discoloration on your skin. But do be cautious. Skin cancer is the most curable of all cancers—with an over 90 percent cure rate—if diagnosed and treated early.

There are three kinds of skin cancers:

1. *Basal cell carcinoma,* the most common skin cancer, originates in the basal epidermal cells. Basal cell carcinoma usually appears as a small, shiny, pearly nodule on the face, neck, hands, or any sun-exposed area. Rare in dark-skinned people, untreated lesions can bleed, crust, and grow down below the surface of the skin to disrupt the normal tissue and even bone. Metastases (spreading of the malignancy) are extremely rare.
2. *Squamous cell carcinoma,* which develops in keratin-forming cells of the epidermal layer. Squamous cell carcinoma usually appears as a red and sometimes scaly lesion that has distinct edges and a central sore that bleeds easily. It is more common on the head and neck areas. Most often found on those with fair skin, it seldom attacks dark people. Squamous cell carcinoma can also develop from premalignant lesions (solar keratoses). Metastases occur in about 1 percent of the cases.
3. *Malignant melanoma,* is the most serious form of skin cancer. Pigment-producing cells called melanocytes give rise to a melanoma, which appears as a dark brown or black molelike growth with irregular borders and irregular pigmentation. Some lesions are multicolored, with red, blue, or gray areas, and the most frequent sites are the upper back and legs. Forty times more cases of melanoma occur on the lower legs of women than on men. About 6,500 deaths each year are attributed to this cancer. The incidence of melanoma in women is second only to lung cancer, and it has been rising lately.

Cancer Treatments

If a biopsy of a lesion indicates cancerous growth you have to consider the options available in treatment. Your dermatologist will make some recommendations based on the extent and type of skin cancer, its location, and your general medical history. The following options are available:

- Electrosurgery—used for the majority of basal cell and small squamous cell carcinomas. It is done using local anesthesia. A curette is used to scrape away the affected tissue, and an electric needle burns away the base of the lesion. The procedure has a 98 percent success rate, usually with good cosmetic results.

- Cryosurgery—the application of icy-cold liquid nitrogen to destroy cancer cells. Appropriate for premalignant lesions and basal and some squamous cell carcinomas, the technique is also performed using local anesthesia; the affected area is frozen, thawed, and refrozen. Cosmetic results are usually good.
- Surgical excision—essential for the removal of malignant melanoma. It may also be used for other skin cancers if your doctor thinks it appropriate.
- MOHS (microscopically controlled surgery)—a technique whereby thin layers of tissues are removed and checked under a microscope, layer by layer, until no more cancer cells can be seen. MOHS surgery is usually performed on stubborn cancers (those that recur), large cancers, and those located in delicate areas such as the corner of the eye. The cure rate is nearly 100 percent but with less satisfactory cosmetic results than other procedures in most cases.
- Radiotherapy—focusing X-ray beams on the skin cancer—is suitable for some cancers of the ears, eyelids, and lips and in the treatment of older patients.

If you have had at least one skin cancer, your chances of developing more are higher than they are for someone who has had none. If you've ever had a skin cancer, see your dermatologist at least twice a year, because early diagnosis is vital.

7

MATCH YOUR SKIN
AND HAIR CARE TO
YOUR CLIMATE

My skin and hair are reliable forecasters of the weather. I can tell if it's going to rain by how limp my hair is. I can tell how cold it is by how chapped my hands and lips are, and my facial skin is a perfect moisture indicator.

Several years ago one of my first patients, an exquisite olive-skinned model, came to see me after an important location assignment. She had found herself off the coast of South America—with uncontrollable hair and oily skin. She was in a panic because she thought her hair and skin had suddenly changed texture. But it was her environment that had changed.

Only in the equatorial depths of the Amazon regions or in the frigidity of the Antarctic are your skin and hair likely to behave consistently. Elsewhere each season brings its own set of health and beauty benefits and problems. Adjust your skin and hair care routines just as you adjust your wardrobe to climate to adapt to climatic fluctuations.

This chapter is composed of two sections. The first section is organized around geographical regions of the United States. The second is organized by season. The idea is to let you see at a glance where you are, and what you can expect in that climate regarding its effect on your skin. If you are planning a trip or relocating to another area, you also should know what to expect.

Matching Your Skin and Hair
to Where You Live and Work

The major regions of the United States show some uniformity of weather conditions within them. This zone guide will help you cope with their climates.

Note: Several cities around the country have hard water, the minerals in which combine with the alkaline salts in some soaps and shampoos to leave a dulling curd on skin and hair. If your area has hard water, avoid alkaline soaps and shampoos and opt instead for synthetic or detergent products.

The Northeast

Cool summers and severe winters with abundant snowfall are characteristic of the north. The mid-Atlantic and coastal areas experience frequent winter storms and well-defined seasonal changes.

Skin Care in the Northeast

The eastern states from Maine to Maryland are industrialized. Concern in the region about acid rain, buried toxic dumps, and other environmental hazards is well founded. Such toxins can and do affect the skin.

Wash your face at least twice daily with a mild, nondrying soap or cleanser; pat dry or air-dry. Oil produced by the skin's oil glands spreads on the surface of the skin during humid spells. This makes makeup vanish and makes your face shiny. Use a mild astringent and oil-absorbing mask to tighten pores.

Hair Care in the Northeast

Autumn days are hard on sun-dried summer hair, and the changes in climate make your hair flyaway and prone to static. If your hair is very dry and unmanageable, rub a bit of olive oil on your palms and work it through the ends of your hair. Don't cut down on the number of shampooings per week; use products designed for a dry scalp, such as deep conditioners.

If you notice an unusual amount of hair loss, don't panic. Autumn (October and November) is the time that the hair naturally thins. It is normal to lose from 80 to 100 hairs, sometimes even more, a day.

Wearing heavy, warm hats protects you from frostbite, but they mat hair and cause scalp perspiration. Always take your hat off when you are indoors, and avoid wearing weather-treated fabrics on your hair—they retard rain and snow, but they act like a scalp sauna.

The Southeast

This region typically experiences hot, humid summers, moderating inland, and mild winters, although it can be cold and wet in the northern sections. There is usually abundant rainfall.

Skin Care in the Southeast

Severe acne is common in the Southeast. It may be partially due to humidity, but more likely it is related to high iodine levels in the soil, which make locally grown food acnegenic. Use moisture-removing absorbing cosmetics such as drying masks, water-based foundations, and loose powders if you have a tendency to shine.

Your chief enemy is the strong sun: Use a sunscreen all year round.

Washington, D.C., is a hard-water area. Avoid alkaline soaps and shampoos there.

Hair Care in the Southeast

From Washington south to the Florida Keys and west to Kentucky, the Southeast can be a humid and difficult place for hair. To cope with high humidity use a strong setting lotion or a mousse.

In the summer keep your hair covered and away from the sun as much as possible. This is especially important for tinted or colored hair, because sun interacts with the chemicals in hair coloring, which causes oxidation and a brassy look.

The Midwest

This region experiences warm summers and cold winters; areas around the Great Lakes have cold winters, heavy snowfall, and hot summer temperatures. There can be extremes of wet and dry, hailstorms, dust storms, thunderstorms, and tornados.

Skin Care in the Midwest

Carry a lip balm with you at all times. Light frostbite when waiting for buses or even walking a few blocks isn't uncommon. It is usually indicated by a very white, numb area on the face. It can also occur on ears, nose, and fingers—and you can have it without being aware of it.

Don't wash your face, shave your legs, or do anything to remove protective oils before going out into the cold. Do cover your skin with a thick oily moisturizer.

Because Minneapolis is a hard-water area, you should avoid alkaline soaps and shampoos if you live there.

Windburn needs nightly treatment. Wash with a mild cleanser and then splash the skin with lukewarm water. The cool water softens and hydrates the skin. Then you must hold the moisture from the water on the skin by applying a light moisturizer and, over that, a thicker oily night cream, concentrating on the wind-whipped areas and the eyes and throat. In severe cases an over-the-counter steroid cream or ointment may be used a few times a day for a few days.

Insect bites and swimmer's itch can destroy summer skin. Poison ivy, poison oak, and poison sumac are rampant throughout the Midwest, and they provoke an allergic reaction in about 70 percent of the population. (If you're allergic to these plants, you'll also be allergic to mango skins, oil from cashew nuts, and a few other obscure plants.) After several contacts you can become so sensitized that, unless it is treated, the itching continues throughout the summer.

Hair Care in the Midwest

The violent weather changes in the middle of the country make hair brittle. If a Minnesota winter can freeze water and make your skin tingle, think of the damage it can do to your hair.

The delicate oils and moisture in your hair strands are vulnerable. Chicago's extremely windy weather is disastrous for hair. Use conditioners that are supplemented with oils and advertized as being "rich" or "deep."

Keep your hair covered at any temperature below 50°F, and keep it uncovered at any temperature above this to avoid a sticky, perspiring scalp.

The Southwest

Summers in the coastal areas are warm, humid, and rainy, but the central areas experience very dry winters and abundant summer sun. The high temperature and low humidity of the desert areas can affect both skin and hair.

Skin Care in the Southwest

If you don't want to look like a western wrangler—leathery-faced and covered with squint lines—sunblocks, moisturizers, and broad-brimmed hats are necessary. Never use a sunscreen with an SPF lower than 15. The incidence of skin cancers in this part of the country is high. (In fact, Tucson has the highest number of cases of malignant melanoma in the United States.) Remember, too, to use sunscreen on your children whenever they go outdoors, starting at six months of age.

The air is pure and clear and often so dry that evaporation of moisture is almost instantaneous. Apply your moisturizer at least a half hour before going out to give it a chance to sink in.

Beware of spicy Texas barbecues; highly seasoned foods bring a flush to the face that can permanently dilate small blood vessels and capillaries if they are consumed too frequently. Keep your face away from camp fires for the same reason. Swimming in icy streams can also promote capillary damage.

Hair Care in the Southwest

Be sure your shampoo and conditioner are suited to the local climate. They should be slightly acidic—that is, with a pH of less than 6.8 (look on the label for the words "low pH")—because there is a high mineral content in much of the water in the region, which makes it hard and can prevent you from having shiny tresses.

The open, relaxed, and informal life-style of the Southwest means outdoor sports and sun-streaked hair. It can also mean brittle, broken ends. An oily conditioner and special split-end treatments with oils can help. Opt also for alcohol-free styling products (one alcohol-free mousse is Revlon's Flex Sun and Sport).

The Northwest

Moderate temperatures along the coast of northern California and rain in all seasons keep the Northwest moist. Much of the climate depends more on altitude than on latitude.

Skin Care in the Northwest

No wonder so many women in the Northwest like the climate so much— it is ideal for skin care. The Seattle area's mist, fog, and moderate seasonal temperature changes are ideal for keeping skin youthful.

Hair Care in the Northwest

In northern California and Oregon and Washington, rain and humidity can make hair limp. If you have trouble making your hair behave, use a spray with alcohol rather than a water base.

Use a hair dryer or even a curling iron to get a smooth effect or to give your hair body. Since your hair is often moist and moist hair is weaker than dry hair, use only a wide-toothed plastic comb. Avoid dragging a brush through tangled hair.

Matching Your Skin and Hair to the Seasons

In most regions of our country the seasons affect temperature, humidity, and wind velocity. With seasonal changes, your skin changes—and so should your grooming routine. It is amazing that women who would never wear a fur coat in July will use the same makeup foundation then as they do in winter. This is a seasonal guide to skin and hair care.

Spring

Skin Care in the Spring

Spring rain and mild temperatures treat your skin and hair kindly. If you've been chapped and parched most of the winter you'll see an improvement in late March, probably before you notice a warming of the temperature. The air gets moister before it gets warmer.

The beginning of spring is a perfect time to get rid of dead dry skin by setting aside an hour or two and steaming your face. (See page 14 for directions on how to steam your skin.) If you look pale or sallow, steam your face over a pot of boiling water into which about a tablespoon of thyme has been added.

Spring is the time for a freshening, tightening, and cleansing mask. Look for one that has a clay body (kaolin should be listed on the label). The clay will absorb some of the skin's moisture, but it will also pick up old cells and absorb oils from slack, enlarged pores. Here are several effective masks:

- MUDD Super Cleansing Treatment (Chattem)
- Sea-Mud Pack (Adrien Arpel)
- Masque Empreinte de Beauté (Lancôme)

Another way of brightening a winter-wan skin is to use a grainy scrub for cleansing. The scrub will remove the sluggish upper layer, and the slight irritation to the skin will bring on a vigorous blood supply to the surface. If you have acne or your skin is prone to bumps, use the grains only to unplug the jammed hair follicles; avoid any massaging motion.

Some scrubs that work well:

- Brasivol Lathering Scrub (Stiefel)
- Buf-Puf Singles (Personal Care Products/3M)
- Exfoliating Scrub (Clinique)

If your skin is thin, dry, and papery, avoid grains and other exfoliators.

It may not feel very warm, but the sun's rays in May are as powerful as they are in July and August, and it is easy to forget how skin-damaging they can be. A spring sunburn will lay down a coat of peeling rather than a basis for a smooth, even tan.

Hair Care in the Spring

Spring hair experiences a period of activity (the fastest and most abundant hair growth is usually in May), but dried and brittle ends are not unusual.

If you like the look of sun-lightened golden highlights in your hair, start using a wash-in lightener or have your hair streaked. But if you prefer it all the same color, protect yourself against sun bleaching by using a natural henna conditioning treatment before spring goes into summer.

Summer

Skin Care in the Summer

When the temperature of the air goes up, the temperature of your skin's surface rises, too. At room temperature the surface of your skin is between 88°F and 93°F. When the room is over 70°F, the sweat glands go into action. When the temperature is over 93°F, you can perspire just sitting still or lying very quietly—perspiration is your body's method of keeping cool. The perspiration and the oil from heat-activated oil glands pour onto your face, coating it with a sticky surface, and you feel less clean. The oil can occlude, or plug, the follicles and thus cause whiteheads. Since perspiration makes pores more likely to occlude, summer is the season for acne formation as well as acne improvement. If you have a tendency to break out on your back and chest, wear natural fibers such as cotton and linen rather than synthetic fibers, which tend to create friction and don't absorb perspiration.

Cleanse more often, but not more vigorously. A cleanser containing salicylic acid—such as SalAc (GenDerm)—will help dissolve the clogs in pores. Use a mild astringent and a clarifier rather than grains to rid the pores of plugs. A product labeled as a clarifier helps somewhat to unplug pores. Finish with a mild astringent (you can make your own by mixing one part vodka with ten parts chilled mineral water). Then set up makeup with a spritz of mineral water.

Light moisturizers, particularly skin gels that are water-based, work well in summer. Try mixing gel rouge with moisturizer before applying.

To remove excess oil from your face after makeup is on, use cotton pads soaked in cold water.

Use all your sun protection knowledge—and use it often. Wear sunblock, sunscreen, and makeup that includes sunscreen in its formula. Use them every day. If anything, skip foundation—but not sunscreen. If your doctor allows you, take two aspirin tablets every morning and every evening for ten days before you venture into the sun. The aspirin will reduce your risk of sun damage. Wear hats with wide brims or visors to protect your face and sunglasses to avoid squinting, which forms lines around your eyes.

Hair Care in the Summer

Sun strips the hair of oils, so if you usually have the greasies only a day after shampooing, you might find your hair more manageable at this time of the year than at any other. One method of keeping hair summerized is to apply hair conditioner before going to the beach or sunning and to leave it on until you leave many hours later. However, this method can result in overconditioning and weakened hair, since the shiny conditioner focuses the sun's rays on your hair, making your head very hot. (If you try this method, afterward wash your hair very thoroughly with two or more shampooings and then rinse with a mild vinegar solution of one tablespoon of white apple vinegar to about one quart water.) Hair gels, designed to add shape and shine, also protect hair. One to try is Estée Lauder's Swiss Control Hair Gel.

Summer means very frequent shampooings, sometimes twice a day. Any shampoo is too harsh under those conditions, but if you wet your hair thoroughly before applying the shampoo and dilute the shampoo slightly with about an equal part of water, your hair should survive the season. Also try using gentle shampoos such as Neutrogena or baby shampoo.

Moisture makes hair swell; heat and humidity can turn a slight wave into a tight curl. You may notice that even perspiration from your scalp can affect your hair's texture. Light hair pomades can help because they prevent the moisture from penetrating the hair shaft.

Summer sun, even if you are careful, can change the color of your hair as well as your skin: Your hair gets lighter and your skin gets darker. For those with golden highlights, that looks great, but if your hair is reddish it can turn an unattractive brassy shade. Coating your hair with a wash-in color close to your own is one way of protecting your natural color.

Some medications, as well as perfumed hair sprays, react with the sun. Avoid lemon rinses, since citrus fruits can spur a photochemical reaction with the sun.

Keep your hair cool while you're out in the sun or even in an after-sport sauna. Hair strands weaken in temperatures over 108°F. Wrap a cold-water–soaked Turkish towel around your hair if you're in the bright sun on a hot day. Brunettes must be especially careful because their dark hair does not reflect the sun's rays and thus will become hotter than blond hair does.

Cover your hair with cream rinse before diving into a swimming pool, and you'll not need a bathing cap—nor will your hair pick up the greenish tinge that comes from copper used in pool-cleaning solutions. Most important, shampoo your hair after pool or ocean swimming and rinse it completely—several times—in pure water.

Fall

Skin Care in the Fall

Summer weekends and vacation sun can leave you with yellowing and dry skin that is plagued by flakes and peeling. Use a superfatted soap and an oily moisturizer on the dry areas.

In autumn facial skin can be both thickened and coarsened from suntanning. You might want to scrub your face with grains or use a soft brush to speed the sloughing off of the outer cells. Use a skin-bleaching cream for general lightening. Over-the-counter bleaching creams include:

- Porcelana (Jeffrey Martin)
- Esoterica (Norcliff Thayer)
- Artra (Plough)

Two reliable products available by prescription are Eldopaque and Eldoquin Forte (both from Elder). For more information on skin bleaches see chapter 23.

In September you may also notice whitish spots on your torso and extremities that are often mistakenly associated with sun exposure. These usually have to do with tinea versicolor, a superficial fungal infection of the skin. Because the fungus acts as a sunscreen, the affected areas don't tan with the rest of your skin and so become more noticeable against a darkened background.

Hair Care in the Fall

Use a conditioning treatment to moisten dry and split ends; hot oil treatments can also ready your hair for winter. Fall is a good time to try a new style, and it is a good season to go bareheaded and allow the air to circulate freely through hair and scalp.

Winter

Skin Care in the Winter

Winter's first cold snap will signal rough going for skin. In summer, heat activates the body systems, and in winter, bitter temperatures slow them down. Your capillaries will constrict and make your face look pale. The skin may become dry, flaky, and raw. (See chapter 2 for a program of help for dry skin.)

Use superfatted soaps on the body and bathe less frequently, for shorter periods of time, and with cooler water. Add bath oils or oilated Aveeno Oatmeal (Cooper). Exfoliate gently about twice a week.

Avoid using very watery moisturizers, which can literally freeze on your face; instead, look for heavier, thicker, oil-based products or products with more active ingredients. Use moisturizer all over the body.

Avoid wearing tweedy woolen slacks or heavy woolen jackets without the proper undergarments. The rough fabric can cause an irritation (wool fibers have tiny "hooks" that can lodge in the skin) because your skin is so dry.

For chapped knees try this:

- Rub your legs and knees with a vegetable oil or an oily cream (Hydrophylic Ointment or Beiersdorf's Eucerin Moisturizing Formula).
- Wrap them in Saran Wrap.
- Cover with a heating pad.
- After about fifteen minutes remove the heat, wrap, and excess cream.

Enough cream will adhere to the skin to avoid painful chapping in this area. If over-the-counter moisturizers don't work, ask your dermatologist for a prescription product.

Don't wash your face or apply a watery moisturizer directly before going out; wait a quarter hour and the protection will be more complete.

Hair Care in the Winter

Use a humidifier if you want to keep your hair in good condition throughout the cold months. Switch to a conditioning shampoo or use a conditioner every time you wash your hair. Deep conditioners should be used once a month. Protective styling mousses will help reduce static electricity.

Moving from room temperature to the outdoors, whether just to your car or for outdoor activity, is very hard on your skin. In the summer the difference between the shade and the sun is seldom more than 15 degrees, but winter is quite different.

A hat is only partial protection for your hair, although it completely protects your scalp. Use a large hat into which you can tuck the ends of your hair. If that is impossible because your hair is long, part your hair and wind it around your neck, and then put it into your coat. A light silk scarf tied babushka style can protect your hair. Or, if you prefer, a loosely knitted cap or snood will save you from brittle split ends.

8

KEEPING YOUR SKIN YOUNG LONGER

When I am asked about aging, I always think of the myth of Eos, the Greek goddess of dawn, who loved a mortal. Fearing that her lover, like other mortals, would die and leave her, she asked Zeus to give him eternal life. Her wish was granted, but Eos had neglected to ask that her lover also be granted eternal youth. Her oversight condemned him to an aging process that would never end. The story reflects the way most of us feel: We want eternal youth rather than just immortality.

If you're lucky and healthy, you'll grow old. Some aspects of aging become apparent very early in life: Our ability to heal, for example, is never as great as when we are babies. Aging begins at birth. And no sooner is maturity reached than a progressive decline in the body's efficiency begins.

What Happens to Skin When We Age

With age the senses become less acute. By age seventy-five, most women have lost two-thirds of their taste buds. Changes in circulation, progressive deterioration of elastic fibers, and a calcifying of fatty deposits within the artery walls are also part of this process.

Skin, too, is subject to several processes of deterioration, beginning in the late twenties and continuing through life:

- Collagen, our skin's "cement," which is responsible for texture and suppleness, becomes cross-linked and degenerates with age.

75

- Elastic fibers responsible for skin resiliency become more abundant, thickened, and cross-linked with age. Calcium salts are often deposited around the elastic fibers, contributing to a lack of elasticity.
- Aging skin is drier than younger skin because of decreased oil, lipid, and sweat production and a lessened ability to retain water. Older women have less oil production than men of similar age.
- Pores become dilated and filled with cell debris (keratin), bacteria, and small hairs. This creates large blackheads (senile comedones).
- The ability to resist small blows without bruising diminishes because skin has thinned and blood vessels are more fragile. (The up side is that older skin does not suffer inflammation with redness and swelling as severely as younger skin does, one reason being that older skin contains fewer blood vessels.)
- The healing process is slower and less effective, so blemishes and flaws remain visible longer. In addition, the skin's ability to resist infections is reduced.
- The cell replacement process in the epidermis slows down, particularly after age thirty-five.
- With the aging of tissue, the yellow pigment lipofuscin accumulates in the dermis, giving the skin a yellowish cast. (Vitamin E taken orally can sometimes counteract this change.)
- Older skin has a decreased ability to generate vitamin D, which is essential for healthy bones. This may lead to fractures of hips, legs, and arms and increased chances of osteoporosis.
- Older skin is more prone to skin cancers and other skin growths.
- The intensity of allergic contact dermatitis decreases with age.

A major determinant of how we age is our individual genetic makeup. However, certain factors can accelerate skin aging, including sun exposure, pollutants, poor nutrition, lack of sleep and exercise, bad habits (drug consumption and smoking), facial expressions, and improper skin care.

Hair and nails are also subject to aging; both grow more slowly as we get older. Decreased blood supplies cause a shrinking of hair follicles and thus a decrease in hair growth. With age, hair also sheds faster, has less pigmentation, and grows smaller in diameter.

Your Skin Aging Calendar

If you are in your late twenties or thirties you probably don't notice how your skin is changing. During these decades the early signs of aging include dilated blood vessels, pigmentary changes, and superficial wrinkles. Moisturizers and sunscreens are essential. Collagen injections may be started.

If you are in your forties or fifties, you probably have become all too aware of your skin's aging. You probably also have started using creams and other emollients to compensate for the slowing of glandular activity that formerly produced natural lubrication. You will notice that wrinkle depth varies from week to week, depending on external factors such as temperature and humidity. Regular chemical peels, collagen injections, perhaps even cosmetic surgery, will help. Have at least one annual skin examination for possible skin cancers.

Fighting Age

Young skin is firm and tight over the underlying body structure. It is also dense and resilient, smooth-toned and even-colored. Science has developed ways to help older women retain or recover these qualities in their own skin. And the search for new methods of retarding the evidence of age goes on.

Recent advances in skin care directed at creating younger skin have been focused on two areas:

1. Building from within—filling in and plumping up the shrinking tissue beneath and in the skin
2. Encouraging skin growth—forcing the skin's natural cell-manufacturing and healing systems to return to a youthful, vigorous, and more rapid schedule so that fresh new cells appear on the surface of the skin and old cells fall away easily

Building from Within

Collagen/Zyderm

In the early 1980s biochemists and physicians experimenting with methods of treating serious burns developed a purified bovine (cattle) collagen, the natural protein found in every part of the body—skin, muscle, tendon, and bone. Collagen fibers in the skin give the body flexibility and form a structure for the growth of new cells and blood vessels; they provide texture, suppleness, and density to the skin. Zyderm collagen was approved by the FDA in 1981.

Zyderm is the brand name for liquid collagen. It comes in the form of a soft white gel that can be injected into the skin to replace tissue lost as the result of age or trauma. Zyderm collagen works below the outer surface to recreate a firm dermis. It replaces lost tissue, becomes part of your own tissue, and like your own collagen, ages naturally. It really is amazing.

Collagen injections can correct small depressions such as scars and wrinkles; they are especially effective in smoothing lines on the forehead and lines around the mouth. Even tiny superficial lines such as those often found around the eyes and on the upper lip are treatable with this kind of procedure.

Zyderm Step by Step

Collagen has been a great success because it is so simple and effective:

The injections take only a few minutes, then the patient can resume her activities immediately. Just three steps are needed:

1. Testing—to be sure that you are not one of the three persons in a hundred who is allergic to collagen. If you are pregnant or suffer from multiple allergies, including to lidocaine, you will be barred from using collagen implants. Don't take antihistamines, salicylates, or steroids for four weeks after the test, as they can suppress a positive reaction.
2. Treatments—usually a series of from two to six half-hour office visits, usually with an interval of two weeks between injections. Using a very thin needle, the doctor will make multiple injections along the line of the wrinkle. There is a sensation of a light scratch along the wrinkle as the injections are given. A slight temporary swelling and blanching occurs after the injection, but there is very little discomfort because Zyderm contains a small amount of the anesthetic xylocaine.
3. Touch-ups—necessary in six to twelve months because Zyderm becomes part of your own tissue and your skin will continue to age. As the aging process continues, additional body mass is lost and must be replaced to keep the skin smooth and plumped up.

After several months, Zyderm is indistinguishable from your natural tissue. It is too early to know the long-term effects, but in more than a dozen years of testing and use it has had a relatively good record. Avoid sunlight immediately after collagen treatments, as well as vigorous exercise, alcohol, and beef and dairy products.

Most disappointments with Zyderm come from underinjecting a wrinkle. Overcorrecting is then necessary because about 30 percent of the Zyderm of each injection, the saline solution and xylocaine portion of it, disappears almost immediately. The overcorrecting is noticeable as a slightly raised area over a depressed wrinkle or scar. An experienced physician knows how to control overcorrecting and undercorrecting. Undercorrecting is more common. The best results are achieved when as much Zyderm as possible is injected as superficially as possible.

Newer Collagen Products

Zyderm II, a more recently introduced improvement, has more collagen and less saline solution in each injection of 1 cubic centimeter. Zyderm II is better than Zyderm I for very deep aging lines and some scars. Zyderm I remains a better choice for fine lines.

A new, longer-lasting collagen product called Zyplast was developed recently. Zyplast is used to correct deeper defects than Zyderm I or II and must be injected deeper into the skin for longer-lasting results. It also can be used for cheek contouring.

Silicone

For more than twenty years a purified form of a synthetic substance called silicone has been used to replace deteriorated or vanishing tissue under the skin's surface. Silicone has an undeservedly bad reputation because of early procedures in which large amounts of liquid silicone were injected into breast tissue. Silicone, unlike Zyderm, can migrate or move from one area to another, and in some early cases this led to embarrassing results. Because silicone is not FDA approved it is not easily commercially available.

Here is a general description of the silicone-injection procedure:

After cleansing the area, minute amounts of silicone are injected with a fine-gauge needle between the dermis and the subcutaneous tissue. (If silicone is injected too superficially, an orange skin discoloration, sometimes permanent, can result.) There are usually three- to four-week intervals between injections. During that time the body recognizes the silicone as a foreign substance; it is not absorbed but becomes surrounded by a shield of connective tissue. Overcorrection with silicone should be avoided because silicone will not be absorbed and corrections will be permanent. Periodic injections are necessary to control developing wrinkles. For example, it takes up to one year to treat nasolabial lines (lines running from nose to mouth) with silicone.

Fibrin and Fibrel

When blood clots form, a protein substance called fibrin is involved. Fibrin foam, a spongelike substance prepared from human blood, has been used as an implant for facial scars since 1957 with excellent results. The foam is actually made from the patient's own blood. But fibrin has never been FDA approved or made commercially available.

In recent years a new fibrin-based treatment for correction of wrinkles and scars has become available. Fibrel—a combination of the patient's own blood, gelatin, and aminocaproic acid (a clotting agent)—stimulates the natural production of collagen at the site of injection. New collagen is deposited at the site of the Fibrel injection; it usually takes three months for the patient's newly formed collagen to replace the injected substance.

As with collagen injections, a test for allergy is necessary before treatment, but a positive skin test occurs in less than 1 percent of all cases. Fibrel is less allergenic and longer-lasting than Zyderm I and II.

The injection technique is similar to that used with Zyderm. The material is injected intradermally until the scar or wrinkle is elevated. The injections are given one or two weeks apart. As with collagen implants, overcorrection is necessary because there is some absorption by the body. Local redness, swelling, burning, and bruising may occur at the site of injection. Fibrel is not FDA approved.

Encouraging New Skin Growth

Plumping the skin from inside can make a dramatic change in your appearance very quickly, but it requires medical assistance. Encouraging new skin growth—so your skin always looks fresh and more youthful—is something you can do on an almost daily basis; it should be part of your own grooming ritual. Abrading your skin to rid the surface of old cells improves your skin's appearance by pushing the younger cells to the surface.

Epidermabrasion/Sloughing Skin

Cell renewal, or the ability of skin cells to grow and replace themselves, is a recent focus of skin care. Methods based on theories of cell renewal work because exfoliation speeds up cell renewal. However, don't exfoliate more than three times a week. Don't exfoliate skin that is extremely sensitive. And never use an exfoliant before going out on a cold, windy day.

Various ways of getting off the old and exposing the new skin are effective:

Mechanical abrasives. Grains, salt, brushes, buffs, and even minerals such as aluminum particles or pumice have been used to gently loosen and rub away the upper layers of skin. Cell production and replacement can be stimulated by removing the upper layer by rubbing, scraping, or filing cells away with:

Grains	Salts	Brushes	Buffs	Sea sponges
Pumice	Apricot shells	Almond	Loofahs	Washcloths

Using such mechanical means of epidermabrasion not only stimulates young cell growth but also increases blood flow, giving skin a fresher look and improving its ability to retain moisture. Exfoliate gently and moisturize immediately afterward.

Chemical peelers. Chemical peelers such as salicylic acid can also work to reveal new skin and encourage skin growth. Milk and yogurt contain lactic acid, a natural moisturizer and skin peeler. (Cleopatra favored this skin-care treatment and took baths in milk.) Some others are:

Citrus fruits	Lemons	Grapes	Papaya
Grapefruit	Apples	Pineapple	Wine

To moisturize and peel your skin, add to your bathwater about a quarter cup of the juice of any of these fruits. If you just want to rinse your face with one of these natural beauty products, use only a tablespoon of the juice to a basin of lukewarm water and be sure to keep your eyes closed when you splash your face. Don't leave any residue of fruit juice on your skin; your final rinses should be clear, pure water.

Masks. Sticky masks capture the old skin cells; when a mask is pulled away, the old cells go with it. Masks that include natural products cleanse the skin and make it look fresher because they rid the skin of its dead, dry upper layer; continued use of these masks can encourage the skin cells to reproduce at a faster rate. Before using any mask, cleanse your face well. Just before applying, touch your face with a terry cloth towel wetted in warm water. Keep the mask on for fifteen to twenty minutes.

Natural Homemade Masks

Here are some simple natural masks that work for many skins. Before you use any product, even a fruit or vegetable mask, test the product on a small dot of your skin to be sure you are not sensitive to the fruit. Many women can eat a particular fruit or vegetable with no problem but develop a reaction to it when it touches their skin.

Cucumber Mask

Cucumbers have a refreshing, bleaching, and stimulating effect. Put one cucumber, peeled, seeded and cut in cubes, into a blender with three ounces of skim or low-fat milk and liquefy. Apply the mixture to your face, neck, arms, and chest as a mask. Allow it to remain ten to fifteen minutes. Wash off and then rinse. You will feel refreshed and your skin will be softened.

Cucumber Lotion

Simply pat the face with cucumber juice and then rinse in cool water.

Strawberry Mask

Wash and hull a handful of fresh strawberries. With a wooden spoon, mash the strawberries into a glass jar (a custard cup works well). Pat the pulp onto your face and neck. Allow it to dry. Then wash clean.

Papaya Rub

Women in the tropics rub their face with papaya fruit to freshen and soften their skin. If you can find a papaya in your market, use the inside of the skin on your face. Papaya is one of the most powerful of the natural skin clarifiers.

Apple Mask

Apples can refresh and rejuvenate skin. Cook one peeled and cored apple in a small amount of milk, mash together, and apply the mixture.

Honey Mask

Honey is good for dry skin. For a mask, mix one tablespoon of honey with either one egg yolk, a few drops of lemon juice, or two tablespoons of milk.

Lemon Juice Astringent

Lemon juice has a bleaching and refreshing effect and is ideal for oily skin. Use the lemon juice straight or mixed with one whipped egg white and a little bit of water. For a lotion that will help tighten pores, mix small pieces of one lemon with an equal amount of vodka and let stand for a week.

Eggs

Egg yolks are good for dry skin. Masks can be made by mixing one yolk with the juice of one lemon, one tablespoon of vodka, and a half cup of sour cream—or with a few drops of olive oil, two grated carrots, and a few drops of lemon juice. Whipped egg whites work on wrinkles and large pores.

Washing Away Old Skin

Many of the products that are used for the treatment of acne also work to freshen aging skin. With acne, peeling is encouraged to loosen plugs of oil. When treating aging skin, the same products peel the skin and make it fresh and new-looking. There is a warning: Older skin isn't as resilient as young skin. Be very gentle, and don't try to rush the peeling. What you'll do is rush a skin irritation.

Some of the acne-treatment products that peel the surface of the skin are:

- Acnaveen Soap (Cooper)—contains oatmeal, which is soothing, and sulfur, a skin peeler
- Acne-Dome Cleanser (Dome)—a mild cleansing paste that is tolerated well even by sensitive skins
- Pernox Scrub (Westwood)—contains sulfur and salicylic acid; can be irritating to dry skin
- Sulpho-Lac (Bradley)—a mild vanishing cream with some sulfur in the compound

Two scrubs that peel skin surface:

- 7-Day Scrub Cream (Clinique)
- Gentle Action Skin Polisher (Estée Lauder)

When using any of these products, be aware of your skin's reaction. You want to encourage new growth, not irritate your skin enough to cause a flaky and inflamed complexion.

New skin is vulnerable to sun and weather conditions. Avoid excess heat, cold, wind, and sun. I am always careful to use a moisturizer containing sunscreen after washing. It protects the surface of my face and I believe it keeps my skin looking soft and fresh longer.

Retin-A

Retinoids are drugs derived from vitamin A; Retin-A (Ortho Pharmaceutical) is the trade name for one of them. Experimentation with vitamin A started long ago when doctors were looking for a cure for acne. After many experiments, retinoic acid, a vitamin A derivative, was developed. Used topically, it was found to be of great help in treating acne. Some patients noticed that skin adjacent to the acne-affected areas that had also been treated with Retin-A seemed much improved in texture and color. The acid, originally used to combat the problems of young skin, was thus found helpful in making older skin look younger and, according to new studies, may even retard skin aging.

How Retin-A Works

Retin-A stimulates the basal layer of the epidermis, where the cells are produced, and accelerates the movement of new and maturing cells toward the surface of the skin, thus speeding up the process of skin renewal, which slows down with age. With the rapid migration of new cells, the old ones are pushed upward and off the skin's surface. The speeded formation of new skin makes the old skin loosen and wash away, exposing a new, younger, and smoother complexion to the world. Concurrent stimulation of the skin's blood supply also makes your complexion rosy.

You need a prescription from your dermatologist for Retin-A. You also need patience and persistence enough to continue to use the product even when a slight irritation develops. Results are usually visible anywhere from three or four weeks to four months after the first application.

Using Retin-A is easy. Use it in the evening, nightly, or every other night at first. (Using it during the day can make your skin more sensitive to the sun.) Retin-A can be applied under, over, or mixed with your moisturizer to minimize dryness.

1. Wash your face and carefully blot it dry or allow it to air-dry. (If it is very dry, use moisturizer after washing.) Wait about thirty minutes before applying Retin-A.
2. Apply the prescribed cream or gel to your skin. Most doctors start with a low percentage of Retin-A to see just how your skin will react. I usually start my patients with the weakest preparation, .05 percent cream. However, your own dermatologist will know what is best for your skin.
3. Gently rub it into the entire area that you want rejuvenated.
4. Allow the Retin-A to remain on overnight; then wash it off in the morning.

If your skin becomes slightly irritated, you know the Retin-A is working. If it is very irritated, however, you may be using too much and should discontinue use for a day or two. The idea is to keep using the acid in a strength that is just under the irritation level. In that way you will keep the skin growing and the skin cells reproducing as fast as possible, yet you will avoid soreness and irritation.

Since Retin-A causes increased sloughing of the epidermal cells, most of which contain pigment, the uneven skin tone typical of aging skin will even out. Even liver spots will lighten. Retin-A also improves the texture of sun-damaged skin by increasing collagen production and making fine wrinkles disappear as deep wrinkles become more superficial. Retin-A also has been shown to eradicate precancerous lesions caused by the sun (solar keratoses) and even to prevent skin cancers. Finally, it has been found to enhance healing—after cosmetic procedures, for example.

There are side effects from using retinoic acid: After a few days' use, retinoic acid can make skin quite sore. The treated areas can become pink, scaly, and very dry. This reaction is most common in women who sunburn easily or have a light complexion and normally very sensitive skin. Make sure to use a milder cleanser and lots of moisturizer immediately after cleansing.

Retin-A makes the skin very sensitive to the sun because it reduces the horny layer by half. Even if you are only taking a short walk on a sunny day, use sunscreen.

After desired improvement is achieved with Retin-A (usually in six months to a year), you should continue use to maintain the improvement. A maintenance program requires using it at least once a week.

5-Fluorouracil

This agent is generally used for treatment of premalignant lesions (solar keratoses) and some superficial malignancies (see chapter 6). However, it also can be used as a modified chemical peel to partially erase wrinkles. The product is available by prescription in a cream or solution form and should only be used under a dermatologist's guidance. Applied once or twice a day for two to four weeks, 5-FU is particularly helpful in the improvement of sun-damaged, rough skin. It seeks and destroys cells, selectively sparing unaffected ones and seeking only those that are sun-damaged.

After an initial angry phase during which a topical steroid cream may help calm and soothe skin, 5-fluorouracil will leave you with smoother, younger-looking skin.

Professionally Administered Chemical Peels—Showing New Skin

Chemical face peels performed by a dermatologist or plastic surgeon are excellent alternatives to surgery for erasing wrinkles and other signs of aging. They are especially effective on sun-damaged skin. A chemical peel can rid the face of some old acne scars, liver spots, tiny lines, and other imperfections.

The process of chemical skin peeling works best on women with fair complexions, for they usually have thin skin and run less risk of the scarring or discolorations that can result when darker skins are involved. However, chemical peels have been used with good results on many women of all complexions.

A chemical peel deliberately damages the skin. Chemicals create a second-degree burn of about the severity of a very bad sunburn. The peel removes the entire epidermis and a portion of the dermis. Until new cells grow to cover the surface, the skin is raw, ugly, and oozing. Results, however, can be quite wonderful.

Chemical Peels Step by Step

Most face peels are done in a doctor's office. The procedures are generally quite similar:

1. The day before the peel, your face is carefully cleansed several times.
2. The day of the peel, your face is cleansed with acetone to remove any oils.
3. The skin is painted with a peel solution using cotton swab applicators. There is a brief burning sensation. A thick white frost forms on the area of peeling.
4. In about a week, the crusty healing mask loosens and reveals new skin. Keeping the area moist will speed healing.

The success of the peel depends on how effective the chemical is in ridding the face of marks and blemishes, and also on how carefully the treated area is blended with the other skin so that there is no line of demarcation. For small-area peels such as a peel on the upper lip, the skill of the physician in feathering and blending the area is crucial.

The new skin is very sensitive, red, and tender (a topical steroid cream will help). It takes several weeks for normal color to return and for the full effects to be seen. At least a week of seclusion is required during the peeling process. (During that time you can meditate on why sunbathing is so damaging for the skin.) Be aware that pregnancy, estrogen-dominant birth control pills, and excessive sun exposure can cause darkening of the peeled areas, especially during the first six months after peeling.

What You Should Know Before Deciding on a Chemical Peel

Chemical skin peels are not without potential problems. Phenol, the chemical most often used for a complete peel, is poisonous and its absorption into the system can cause kidney damage. For this reason, phenol should not be used on people suffering from liver, kidney, or heart disorders. In addition, there is always some possibility of scarring, especially at the jaw near the neck. (The neck is never peeled, because it usually scars.)

Tiny white cysts called milia often appear on a peeled face about a month after the procedure. They can be persistent and can be removed by a dermatologist. Pigmentary discolorations and bacterial and viral infections (herpes) may also appear.

As with all new skin, shield a chemically peeled face from the sun. The very best time for a peel is late autumn or midwinter.

Trichloroacetic Acid (TCA)

There are less dramatic and less traumatic methods of chemically peeling skin than by using phenol. Trichloroacetic acid has been used for many years to peel the upper layers of the skin to reveal new skin. The less concentrated the acid, the more shallow the peel and the shorter the healing time.

The procedure is very similar to a phenol peel. The face is cleansed of facial oils and the acid (no more than a 20 to 35 percent solution for a light peel) is applied to the skin with cotton swabs. The acid is left on the skin for about one minute. If left on for longer than two minutes, a stinging and burning sensation will occur. The treated area may or may not turn white, depending on the concentration used.

In about three days the old skin will peel. The new skin will look newer and fresher. This treatment refreshes the skin but does not erase deep wrinkles. It is also too mild to rid the skin of deep discolorations. However, light brown spots will disappear and large pores will look smaller. The advantage is that TCA is suitable for use on the delicate skin of the neck, and it will not cause scarring. TCA treatment can be done every two weeks to refresh skin and improve its texture.

Professional Dermabrasion

On a single day last year I consulted with two patients who had very different skin types and different complaints, and I gave them both the same advice: Consider dermabrasion. One was a woman in her thirties whose cheeks were covered with depressed scars caused by acne. The other woman was almost twenty years older; her skin was weather-beaten, brownish, and discolored.

Skin planing, or dermabrasion, though originally developed to eliminate acne scars, has been used for various cosmetic and medical purposes. Dermabrasion de-epidermizes the skin; everything above the dermis is destroyed. The procedure can be used to erase fine wrinkles and brownish discolorations or other changes of the aging skin. A skilled physician is the key to success. Dermabrasion can be combined with collagen injections or chemical peels.

What Happens During Dermabrasion?

Dermabrasion grinds away the epidermal layer of the skin with a very fine sanding process. Diamond-coated instruments (fraises) have made great improvements in the procedure possible.

You are usually asked to arrive at the doctor's office at least an hour before the surgery and to wear button-on rather than pullover clothing. You may also want a friend to be on hand to accompany you home, since you will be medicated during the procedure.

1. A sedative is administered to relax you and help you feel a bit sleepy.
2. The area to be dermabraded is cleansed and may be painted with an antibacterial solution.
3. The area is then frozen with a freezing spray. Local anesthetics are often used.
4. While the skin is held taut, the surgeon abrades the skin in segments to the depth required to rid the skin of scars or marks.
5. A special dressing of synthetic membrane is applied. The planed surface is moist and tends to ooze. It develops a crust in about twenty-four hours after the procedure and generally looks terrible. You'll probably need to take pain-killers for a day or two as well.

After the procedure, ten to fourteen days may pass before you will feel comfortable in public.

The skin that grows back is very sensitive. It remains red, tender, and easily irritated for several months; it is essential to protect it from ultraviolet rays of the sun. Some women with dark complexions have a tendency to hyperpigmentation (darkening of the skin).

You should be aware that dermabrasion is traumatic and can trigger an outbreak of herpes or other stress-triggered skin problems. The procedure is also not advised for anyone with warts, burns, or tendency to keloidal scarring.

How to Disguise a Red Face

Chemical peels, 5-fluorouracil treatment, and dermabrasion will leave you with reddened skin for some time. This is what you can do to help you get through this period:

• Use a green base under your makeup to camouflage redness. Some examples are Velluto Liquid Toner Verde (Borghese), Porcelain Cover Base (Adrien Arpel), and Tuna Cover Base (Countess Isserlyn).
• Effective heavier concealers include CoverMark (Lydia O'Leary) and Continuous Coverage (Clinique).

The procedures touched on in this chapter are all regularly used with some success by hundreds of thousands of people. They often change lives, giving the patient a new way of seeing herself and changing the way she is perceived by others.

9

LAVISH ATTENTION TO
PACKAGING PAYS OFF

A recent study shows that when people meet someone new, the first thing they notice is the face. That is true for men 34 percent of the time, for women 27 percent of the time. Clothes, hair, and other features are less critical than the face to the forming of that all-important first impression. The conclusion is obvious: To prepare for any meeting, your face must look its best. How is that to be managed? Cosmetics.

Cosmetics that marry chemical technology with fashion can add years of youthful elasticity to your skin and can form a shield between your skin and the outside world. The challenge is finding the right product for your skin texture, and color that enhances your personality and distracts from any less than perfect features. Given the thousands of products on the market, this is no small task.

I use cosmetics—moisturizers, foundations, lip and eye products. They make me look and feel better and help me function more effectively. I am continually experimenting with new cosmetics, partly because of curiosity and partly because novelty is a joyful experience.

Cosmetic products, techniques, and expert advice once available only to the rich are now available in most department stores and even in small drugstores. Thousands of products have been formulated that will:

- Enhance their wearer's appearance
- Act as a protective barrier against potential skin problems
- Provide therapeutic treatment for minor skin blemishes. (So many of

the new cosmetics include ingredients designed to benefit the skin that, if you choose properly, you can easily have cosmetics with some therapeutic value.)

According to the Food and Drug Administration, a cosmetic is a substance that is intended to be rubbed, poured, sprinkled, or sprayed on, introduced onto, or applied to the human body for cleansing, beautifying, or promoting attractiveness. Real scientific advances in cosmetics have been made during the past few years; today the industry receives fewer than one customer complaint for every 100,000 users of hair, skin, and makeup products. Every cosmetic made by a major company undergoes rigorous testing before reaching the marketplace.

Most companies use special terms to describe the qualities of their products and attract consumers:

- *Hypoallergenic* means less likely to cause allergic reactions.
- *Noncomedogenic* products are those that a company feels will not encourage blackheads or whiteheads.
- *Dermatologist-tested* indicates that a physician supervised or helped organize the tests.
- *Clinically tested* indicates that the tests were done under strict supervision.

Six Rules for the Use of Cosmetics

Every so often you may find your skin red, tight, or bumpy after using a new product. Such a reaction is inevitable if you have broken one of the six rules for avoiding adverse reactions and receiving the full benefits of the products:

1. Read all cosmetic labels carefully and follow directions exactly until you are familiar with the product and your reaction to it. Know something about your own sensitivities, and note any chemicals that have affected you adversely.

2. Test new cosmetics for possible allergic reactions:

- Apply a small amount to the inside of your forearm.
- Leave it untouched for about twenty-four hours.
- Check for redness and blisters.
- If itching, stinging, burning, or redness results, you would be wise to throw the product away—no matter how expensive it was.

"Hypoallergenic" on the label does not mean trouble-free. The prefix *hypo* means "less"—less in the way of allergens and irritants—but none of the makers of hypoallergenic cosmetics can agree exactly on what ingredients make a product less sensitizing. Most cosmetics made by reputable cosmetic manufacturers, whether hypo or not, have been formulated to avoid complications. "Fragrance-free" on the label is usually a plus, since it means a cosmetic includes one fewer ingredient that can cause trouble. However, some so-called fragrance-free or unscented products contain masking odors to cover the base odor, so a reaction may still be possible. If you suspect a reaction to any product, stop using it immediately. The longer you use it, the more severe the reaction can become. You seldom "get used to" an allergen; in fact, you increasingly lose an ability to tolerate it. In some cases a few ingredients in different products can enhance each other and together act as an allergen.

3. Wash your hands and rinse them well before applying any cosmetics. Bacteria and viruses can be carried to the eyes, nose, and mouth.

Never use another person's cosmetics; avoid testers at cosmetic counters. If you want to learn the techniques of a makeup artist, try bringing your own cosmetics with you (which is not really what they'll want, since they usually hope to show you the effects of new colors) or insist on the use of throwaway applicators.

4. Store cosmetics carefully. Close the container of each cosmetic carefully after using it. Doing so protects the water and oils in the cosmetic formulas from evaporation and deterioration and increases their longevity. Buy only the smallest possible quantity. If you are stocking up on a cosmetic, buy two small sizes rather than the large size. Store cosmetics in cool, dark places. The freshness of the product makes a difference. Close-outs and final sales on some cosmetics are often a waste of money for the same reason. The cases are seldom airtight, and an old lipstick may well be dried and uneven before your first application.

If your cosmetic products have changed color or the texture is different from when you bought them, it is time for replacement. This is especially true of eye and lip products, which, if contaminated or outdated, can invite infection.

To keep your cosmetics fresh and color-true as long as possible, especially natural formulations containing foodstuffs, store them in lightproof containers in your refrigerator. The vegetable crisper is pefect. Do *not* store any cosmetics in the freezer.

5. Demand the best. Cosmetics are not going to change your life or make you happy—but they should make you look terrific or they are not worth it, no matter what you pay. Keep only the best (not necessarily the most expensive) next to your skin.

Do not be intimidated by sales pitches, mesmerized by packaging, or lured into a fantasy world by color photographs of flawless beauties. Beautiful models have skin problems, too—photographic retouchers are usually more important to their look in the ads than the products the models recommend. You can select products from various manufacturers if you prefer to mix brands. Do not hesitate to do so. However, use products only for the areas for which they are recommended.

6. *Apply all cosmetics gently.* Irritations can be caused by the way you apply cosmetics as well as by the ingredients in the products. Be gentle to avoid irritating your skin; use feathery light strokes and select products that blend easily. Avoid scratching or dragging your skin with pencils or rasping it with stiff brushes.

Irritation caused by a product or improper use of a product appears almost immediately, but an allergic reaction doesn't appear until you have used the product several times. When this happens, the products are naturally suspect, but don't forget to consider the applicators, especially if the products involved are for the eyes. I have seen many more women allergic to mascara brushes than to mascara. (For more about allergic reactions see chapter 19.)

How to Read the Labels on Skin-Care and Makeup Products

Here is a key to the function of ingredients commonly listed on cosmetics labels:

- Emollients—vegetable and mineral oils, lanolin, silicone, isopropyl myristate
- Emulsifiers—lanolin, lecithin
- Humectants (hold moisture to skin)—glycerine, propylene glycol, sorbitol
- Thickeners—cellulose gums
- Preservatives—alcohols, parabens (propylparaben and methylparaben), aldehydes, sorbic acid, potassium sorbate, quaternium 15, imidazolidinyl urea, phenyl mercuric acetate
- Antioxidants—vitamins A, C, D, and E
- Chelating agents (prevent discoloration)—EDTA (ethylene diamine tetra-acetate)
- Fragrance/flavor—musk, saccharin (found in lipsticks)
- Colors—iron oxides, carmine, titanium dioxide
- Sunscreens—UVB sunscreens: PABA, PABA esters, padimate, cinnamates, salicylates; UVA sunscreens: oxibenzone or benzophenone compounds, anthranilates
- Waxes (increase viscosity)—paraffin, beeswax, carnauba, ceresin, candelilla
- Fatty alcohols—cetyl alcohol, stearyl alcohol
- Additives—collagen, elastin, allantoin, sodium RNA, oil of turtle
- Fillers (compressing agents)—talc, kaolin, silicates, magnesium carbonate

A Toner by Any Other Name . . .

A woman should tone her skin before applying makeup—after washing, rinsing an endless number of times, and patting dry. This step is easily overlooked and frequently forgotten, but it can make the difference between makeup that stays on and makeup that vanishes. The oilier the skin, the higher the alcohol content in the toner should be.

A toning lotion is designed to make the skin look fresher, remove cleanser residue, and make the pores less noticeable. The toners include fresheners, astringents, and clarifiers. The terms *toner, freshener, astringent, clarifying lotion,* and *pore lotion* are often used interchangeably. There is no standardization of names. To tell which product you are buying (or using), read the label and notice where the ingredients appear on the label (the nearer the top of the list, the higher the percentage of the ingredient).

Fresheners. The operative ingredient in a freshener is alcohol, and it is very drying. To make the skin feel cool and refreshed, fresheners usually are high in alcohol and include a dash of menthol or camphor. Fresheners are ideal for use in the tropics or for very oily skin. If you have combination skin, using a freshener on just the nose or the central oily area of the face (the T-zone) can normalize the area and provide a good base for makeup.

Astringents. The operative ingredient in an astringent is alum, aluminum sulfate, chloride, or acetone, all of which mildly swell the skin around the pores to make the pores appear smaller. These products also usually include a small quantity of alcohol.

Some astringents are marketed under the buzz words *pore lotion,* but a check of the ingredients will usually reveal aluminum salts in a watered down low-alcohol solution. You can get the same effect by mixing a bit of liquid antiperspirant in water or witch hazel. Or mix about a teaspoon of alum (available on the spice shelves in some supermarkets or in your pharmacy) in a small jar of witch hazel.

Nothing that feels bad is necessarily good. Some products include rubifacients that irritate the skin and redden it. When the skin is irritated it will puff slightly and your astringent will seem to work well. Tingling, itching, tightness, and a drawing-in feeling tell you that your astringent or freshener is too strong or is irritating. If you wish to continue to use the product, apply it with a cotton ball that has been moistened in water. Mix astringent and water this way until you get the fresh feeling you want without any irritating sensations.

Clarifiers. The operative ingredient of clarifying lotion whisks away dead skin. To make the skin look brighter and clearer, the lotion contains a keratolytic agent that breaks down the keratin in the upper layer of the epidermis to remove dead cells. The agents commonly used are salicylic acid, resorcinol, or benzoyl peroxide. Some clarifiers are extremely alkaline and others have a high alcohol content; these are not for women with sensitive skin. A clarifying lotion is closer to an exfoliant than to an astringent.

Recommended Skin "Toners"

- Tonique Douceur (Lancôme): contains no alcohol
- Clarifying Lotion (Clinique): This comes in various strengths and is my personal favorite.
- Mild Action Protection Tonic (Estée Lauder)
- Skin Sense Clarifier (Molton Brown)
- Skin Sense Tone (Molton Brown): comes in two strengths
- Witch hazel: If you add some perfume to change the smell, it works as well as many commercial toners.

Moisturizers—Protection at Its Best

Moisturizers, night creams, and body lotions are similar: They are mostly oil-in-water emulsions. After the water evaporates it leaves behind a thin, even layer of oil and humectants and, if the product is perfumed, some perfume oils. Some moisturizers contain a special anti-irritant such as allantoin; others feature special oils or herbal extracts; still others contain vitamins that will not affect deficiencies in the body but may improve failing skin functions.

Moisturizers come in the form of hand creams, moisture creams, and lotions. Variations in the medium do not significantly change the product's effects.

Moisturizers are designed to spread a thin film on the surface of the skin. After an application, the skin should feel soft, moist, flexible, and smooth, with no tacky or waxy feeling. Every woman needs a moisturizer, regardless of her skin type. Most women prefer a light moisturizer that is mostly water, especially for daytime use. Lotions are usually lighter than creams or ointments.

Which Moisturizer Is Best for You?

The wrong moisturizer can prevent even the most perfect foundation from adhering to your skin, and too much of even a good product can have the same effect. If your makeup fades, smudges, or vanishes within a few hours of application, do not throw out your expensive foundation until you first switch moisturizers to see if a different product under the foundation will help. Change your moisturizer when you change your seasonal clothes—in the spring and in the fall:

- Summer moisturizers should be watery. In a moist summer climate, select a moisturizer that includes a humectant such as glycerine—it will draw moisture from the air to the surface of the skin.

- Winter demands an oily product; with too much water, a moisturizer can actually freeze on the face and provide no protection for dry, chapped skin.

Would you wear a heavy coat in the summer? A light blouse in the cold? Protect your skin and it will better protect you. I always urge my patients to start fresh as the seasons change. Use your favorite products, add some new colors, and remember to consider texture as well as color and tone.

Foundations

A foundation should do as much as possible to create the illusion of a perfect skin. It also provides protection: Whether you are in the sun, an air-conditioned office, or outdoors, your foundation is a vital protection for your skin. It acts as a shield and safeguard against wind, sun, and pollutants.

Foundation textures include liquid, cream, stick, cake, tube, and mousse. The best texture for you is the one you can apply most easily and over which you feel you have most control. Most women prefer liquid, and most apply it with their fingers.

Water is the basic ingredient in most liquid and cream products. Other ingredients include oils, waxes, colorants, emulsifiers, and humectants. If you want a true water-based foundation, look for a lotion that will separate and must be shaken before each use. (One such is Clinique's Pore Minimizer Makeup.) That sort of product is essentially a pigmented powder in a light, watery astringent. You can actually make a reasonable foundation just by mixing a small quantity of moisturizer with about a teaspoon of powder.

Read your labels to get the effect you want; *dewy, moist,* and *glowing* mean an oil-based foundation; *matte, smooth,* and *flawless* are buzz words for water-based foundations, which usually contain oil-absorbing ingredients such as clay and zinc oxide. Dry skin needs a thick oil-based foundation that will hold and add moisture. Combination skin may require using two different foundations.

If you don't routinely use sunscreen, make sure that your foundation or moisturizer contains a sunscreen. Two foundation products that contain extra sun protection are Teint Extreme Protection Creme Makeup (Chanel) and Active Protection Makeup with Sunscreen (Max Factor).

Cosmetics with vitamin E included will to some degree prevent UV light–induced skin damage.

Applying the Foundation

You can never really tell if a foundation, your most important makeup, is wrong for you until it is too late. Usually the product must be worn several hours before you know if it is right for you.

To apply:

1. Dot on foundation in the midsection of your face.

2. Using the dots as little wells, continue to dot outward and upward toward, but not into, the hair line.
3. When applying any cosmetic to the eye area, use only the fourth (ring) finger—it's the weakest—and then dot very gently.
4. Do not rub, stroke, or move the skin in any way.

After you have applied the foundation, study your face to see if there are any areas that need extra coverage or that are too dark or too light. A dab or two of a lighter or darker shade can then be applied and patted in to blend well. Do not forget eyelids, under the tip of your nose, your chin, or your earlobes if you have an off-the-face hairstyle.

For flawless coverage:

1. Apply a very thin coat of foundation.
2. Allow it a minute or two to dry.
3. Dampen your face with a natural or small-pored sponge and apply a second thin coat. (Triangular sponges are easy to use.)

To select the right shade:

• Ruddy or florid skin—select a beige with a greenish undertone.
• Olive or yellowish skin—select a beige with a pink or coral tone.
• Mature skin—a tone that is more pink than beige is best.
• Black skin—select a foundation with rust or wine highlights to counter green and blue undertones.
• If you have brown spots, a foundation with a lavender tone will help. If you have uneven skin color, a white primer under the foundation will even the tone.
• If you work in an area under fluorescent lighting, use a slightly rosier tone than your skin, as this type of lighting washes away color.

To get the closest color match possible test a foundation on the side of your cheek or on your jawline; the skin on the inside of the wrist or your hand usually doesn't have the same color or oil glands your face has.

You can change the color of your foundation with the seasons or for different occasions. For example, a paler version of your foundation is attractive for evening makeup and under dimmer lights.

Concealers

Nobody is perfect. That's why concealers were invented. These products are skin-colored creams or crayons that disguise and camouflage by using the optic principles of light and shadow. Light makes an area seem closer, larger, and therefore emphasized; a dark shade makes the same area smaller and farther away, less conspicuous.

Concealers are used to create artificial lights and shadows on the face; they can minimize flaws, create symmetry, and make blemishes appear to vanish. But because they are a different texture from the foundation, they are tricky to use and require deftness and skill in application and blending.

Some skin problems require opaque foundations to disguise them. These concealers work quite well for blemishes or imperfections that are flat—conditions such as broken capillaries and spider veins, skin discolorations, port wine birthmarks, and freckles (see chapter 23). Opaque makeup products are available in waterproof formulations and a broader range of shades from ivory to brown. Two good products are Covermark (Lydia O'Leary) and Dermablend Cover System (Dermablend).

How to Resculpt Your Nose

The shape of one's nose is a common source of dissatisfaction, partly because it is the first thing we see in the mirror every day other than our eyes. Very few of us are born with perfect nose proportions, and our noses usually become even less attractive with age. Rhinoplasty, a "nose job," is a commonly done cosmetic surgery procedure. However, several common complaints can be corrected with cosmetics.

You need a foundation or concealer that is two shades darker than your natural skin color foundation plus another foundation or concealer a shade or two lighter than your natural skin color. Use these two colors to sculpt your nose as follows:

- Uncentered nose—move it visually by drawing a light line slightly off center in the direction you want to "move" your nose.
- Bump—apply a dark sculpture over the area and blend carefully.
- Too long—visually shorten by darkening the nose from a point even with the bottom of your upper eyelids to the brows. Shorten the bottom by darkening the tip.
- Large or long tip—lift by applying light color on the tip of the nose to midbridge.
- Bulbous end—carefully darken the nostril area (the side and the tip of the nose) and lighten the top with a line that goes from the end toward the bridge to give the nose a narrow effect.
- Too wide—narrow with dark shading on the sides for the entire length.

Then gently apply regular foundation over this base.

How to Conceal a Concealer

Concealers are the most difficult of all makeups to apply well. Check your efforts in natural light and from several angles. Use a fine sable brush to apply a concealer if you find you tend to get too much on, and then use your clean fingers or the tip of a soft sponge to blend well.

- *For large areas* (over a square inch): Use over the moisturizer and under the foundation so the concealer can be controlled and placed only where needed. This seems to work best for large areas such as the sides of a too-broad nose or too-full cheeks and to hide nasolabial (nose-to-mouth) creases.
- *For small areas* (as when hiding bright red blemishes): Dot the concealer under and over the foundation and blend to conceal the demarcation.
- *For over a blemish:* With acne-prone skin avoid applying an oily concealer over a blemish. Use medicated acne makeup for that purpose, even if you find the product too drying for general use. (Cleargram/Young Pharmaceuticals, Liquimat/Owen, Acne-Aid lotions/Stiefel and Anti Acne Control Formula/Clinique are four such products.)

Powder

When your foundation is perfectly applied and your concealer is blended well, the final set of preparations to enhance your features is the application of powder. Powder acts as a veil and a primer; it is drying and will set the oils and water in other cosmetics so they stay in place. Powder comes in various forms, but talc, clay, oil-blotting agents, and colorings are the basic ingredients of all of them. Women who don't like using foundation can apply a pressed powder in a shade that matches skin tone over their moisturizer.

Some powders change color after they have been mixed with natural oils on the skin, so you may have to experiment to find one that is right for you. Translucent powders are ideal for oily skin. My favorite powder is Clinique's Transparent Face Powder.

Brushes, puffs, and pads are used to apply the powder as evenly as possible. For a light dusting, just to add a matte finish to the foundation, use a brush and work inward—opposite the way you applied the foundation. Don't use too much of the powder; it can cake up.

To make sure your powder stays on, use a powder puff of a velvety material and blot the powder onto the face, then use cotton or a soft brush to whisk away any excess. (A fluffy lamb's wool or cottonball puff is harder to control.) Your powder should last at least four hours. Women with oily T-zones may need to touch up with powder a few times a day.

Translucent powder controls shine and reflects more light than other powders. It does not contain titanium dioxide or zinc oxide, as full coverage powders do. The thicker the coating, the less transparent the powder. Match the powder as closely as possible to the skin on your neck. Too many women wear rosy or tan powders matched to their cheeks and the result is an obvious line of demarcation near the jaw.

A professional tip: Mix powder with baby talc (half and half) in a small glass. Then strain it through a stretched hose. This helps to keep the powder sheer and light.

Allergy alert: Perfumes and starches in powders can cause allergic reactions. If you sneeze when applying your powder or are bothered with a runny nose while applying your makeup, switch to cornstarch for a short time and see if the allergy disappears.

Finding the Right Shade of Powder

Select powder shades that blend well with your foundation and complexion:

- For sallow or pale skin, look for a slight lavender tone that will warm your skin; avoid rust shades that will look aging and dirty.
- For olive or yellow-toned skin, pink and cream tones will be best.
- For florid or ruddy faces, look for a greenish or gold tone.
- For black skin, choose rust and tan colors without blues or greens, and be sure your powder is dark enough so that there is no ashy or dry look to your skin.

Blusher (Rouge or Contour)

The healthy glow associated with exercise and well-being comes in the form of cheek-coloring pressed powders, pastes, creams, liquids, and gels. *Rouge* is an old term for iron oxide, a reddish powder used in polishing gems and metals that was once also the basis for most cheek colorants. (Iron oxide is still a significant component in most products designed to add color.) Most cream blushers are pastes with a wax or oil base; most gels have a petroleum jelly base. The longest-lasting colors are in powder form. All products contain preservatives; some include perfumes.

Why use a blusher? A dab of lipstick blended and worked into the skin would also provide color, but lipstick is hard to control, and the dragging of the sticky lip color across your cheeks is messy. Powder products applied with a soft brush usually work best with an oily complexion, and cream products applied with fingers or a damp sponge usually work best with dry or older skin. People with a deep or highly colored complexion can use a gel, but gels are difficult to apply evenly. They have a tendency to dry very rapidly and leave no time for blending. Crayons and pencils are excellent in theory, but blending in their coloring is difficult in practice.

Blushers do more than apply color. Because of the optical illusion that color makes possible, blushers also form contours. How and where the blusher is applied is as important to the final effect as the shade and tone of the product. To achieve the best results with a powder blush you need a good brush (those that come with the products are often difficult to control).

How to Reshape Your Features with Blusher

A general rule is to offset any weakness of your facial features: Rounded faces are treated with vertical dark strokes; narrow faces are played up with light.

- If your jaw is too wide, narrow your face by applying your blusher low on your face parallel to your nose and mouth, and blend it into the wide jaw line.
- If your jaw is too narrow, keep your blusher high on your face, making sure no color is lower than your nostrils.
- If your face is too round, brush with a diagonal stroke from your temple almost to your mouth, and then blend toward the ears.
- If your face is too long, visually "cut off" the top and bottom by brushing color on the tip of your chin and the top of your forehead. Keep the color running horizontally across your face.

Always use a light touch and blend well.

Selecting the Blusher for Your Skin Tone

Blushers come in various colors. When choosing a blusher take into account both the color tone of your foundation and your own skin tones. A light bright pink looks sickly on a dark complexion, and a rust looks like a dirty streak on light skin. Blondes and women with ash-brown hair and light skin coloring or silvery hair can use pink and rosy tones in their blusher. Women with sallow complexions should look for a lilac or coral hue. Women with black skin should select rusts and spice colors.

You can get a very natural effect by using a light color first and then a darker shade of the same color family on top as a finish.

In tribal societies painting the face and body probably evolved as a charm against evil, and later the designs that women used identified them as members of a social group or tribe. It has not changed much. Makeup still serves as a banner: When you put on your makeup you assume a public persona.

10

THE EYE-DEAL WAY TO
LOOK AND BE SEEN

If I were shipwrecked on a desert island and could take only one product, I would not take eye shadow or mascara. I would take sunscreen. But since I am here and can enjoy a vast array of cosmetics—as many as I feel make me look and feel spectacular—I am rarely without eye makeup.

Color applied to the upper lids has been a basic part of makeup since the Egyptians first developed the practice as protection against the sun. Eye shadow can benefit your health, since it deflects the sun's burning ultraviolet rays from the thin, vulnerable skin of the eyelids. Once you start wearing eye shadow, you do not feel really dressed without it.

Tea Therapy

Eyes normally produce enough liquid to keep them clean and healthy. If you want to give your eyes a special treat after being out in the sun, soak two balls of cotton in iced tea and apply to shut eyes. Then lie down, your feet higher than your head, and you will soon feel bright-eyed again. Try this when your eyelids are burned and tender—the tea soothes the parched skin very quickly.

Avoiding Eyestrain

To keep your eyes in good condition and ready to benefit from cosmetics, be sure you protect them from strain, glare, dust, and dirt. Avoid reading, writing, or close work in poor light, and take a break from computers or word processors every few hours to refocus your eyes on a distant object. Do not read anything on slick reflective paper when in bright sunlight, and wear sunglasses to shade your eyes from glare.

Eye Savers

Tears are your eyes' first defense; they dilute and carry away any substance that enters or irritates the sensitive whites of the eyes or their visual windows, the corneas. Avoid rubbing your eyes; when they are itchy, wash them out with cool water. For frequently itchy eyes, be suspicious of hair spray, hair dyes, nail polish, eyebrow bleach, shampoos containing formaldehyde, or any cream you apply over your face or hands. Mascara and even eyedrops are excellent growth mediums for some bacteria and molds, and infections can be mistaken for an allergic reaction. If you rub your itchy eyes, you run a chance of spreading an existing infection.

Eye cosmetics are more rigorously tested and regulated by the FDA than any other type of cosmetic product. Unless you suffer from a specific allergy, most products are safe to use. If an eye cosmetic does get into your eyes, a flush of artificial tearing solution such as the following will rid your eye of the problem:

- A/K Rinse (Akorn)
- Lavoptick Eye Wash (Lavoptick)
- Refresh (Allergan)
- Water with a tiny dash of salt in solution (less than one-eighth teaspoon per cup of water)

The thin skin of the eyelids is very prone to dryness and wrinkles. When applying any eye makeup never drag the skin. Keeping eyeliner pencils in the refrigerator with other cosmetics will prolong their life and keep their colors pure, but a cold pencil is hard. If you find your pencil too hard, simply warm its tip in your hand. When removing eye makeup use a product made especially for the job, or a facial cleanser if the label says it can be used around the eyes. Use your fingers to work the cream outward over the eyelids, toward the outer corner and then inward toward the nose. Blot away with soft tissues and rinse.

Note: If eyes are teary, bloodshot, or painful, see an ophthalmologist. If there is a problem with eyelids, see a dermatologist. (For more about eye care see chapter 20.)

You and Your Shadow

You will need several "tools of the trade" when you are applying eye makeup. Brushes, Q-tips or other cotton swabs, small rubber-tipped smudgers, and eyelash curlers all have a job to do. Be sure they are clean and dry each time you use them.

Avoid irritating ingredients in your eye shadow. Carefully check the ingredients in any product you use to be sure it is free of mercury. If you encounter a product that makes you feel itchy and leaves your lids swollen and angry, switch colors. The irritation might come from the pigment rather than the cosmetic base. Plum and violet tones seem to be more irritating than blues and browns. Try switching products, too—from powders to creams, for example.

Powder products usually have more depth, cover, and cling than cream products. This is because the pigments in powders are more concentrated. (Lip pencils have more intense pigments than lipstick for a similar reason.)

Powdered eye shadows are similar in composition to pressed powder. They include kaolin, zinc stearate, and an anticaking ingredient, and the colors are usually chemically compounded. Powder lasts longest and works well on oily lids. Apply it with a small brush rather than the little sponge provided in the case, but do not throw away the sponge covering to the powder—it protects the powder and keeps it clean.

Liquid and cream eye shadows are water-based with thickeners and emulsifiers, waxes, perfumes, and colors. They are best for older, drier lids.

Applying Eye Shadow

Magazines have full-page advertisements promoting the use of three or more colors to create beautiful, butterfly-like eyes, and shadows are sold in colorful arrays of matched shades. It takes time and patience to master the skills of using them. Three shades of the same color are usually sufficient to get a dramatic effect.

To make sure your eye shadow stays where you put it, resists gathering in any creases on your lids, and lasts as long as possible, first apply foundation, then powder to your eyelids. Although the modified oil glands of the eyelids don't supply much natural oil, constant movement in the eye area wears off any cosmetic, so your eye makeup needs to be checked during the day. (You can also try an eye makeup base, such as Elizabeth Arden's Eye-Fix Primer.)

How to Reshape Your Eyes with Shadows

Use light, medium, and dark shades in the following way:

- *Prominent lids that look puffy:* De-emphasize the prominence with medium to deep shades, and create a geometric illusion to minimize roundness. Highlight with a light shade under the brow and a medium or deep shade on the lid. Extend shadow from the inner corner to the center.

- *Small eyes:* Apply a pale shadow all the way from the lashes to the brows. Smudge a darker shade along the crease line. Be generous with mascara.
- *Close-set eyes:* Apply a tiny dab of pale highlighter shadow between the inner eye corner and the bridge of the nose, and use the same shade under the brow. A medium shade goes from the center of the lid outward, slightly past the outer edge of the eye.
- *Deep-set eyes:* Use two shades of the same color. Color the lid and under the brow with a medium color. Color the crease with a light color.
- *Wide-set eyes:* Define the shape of the eyes by using a medium tone on the inner part of the lid and from the inner corner of the eye to the brow. Use a light color on the outer edges.

Eyeliner

Now that you have applied eye shadow, add accent and definition with your eyeliner—either liquid, pencil, or cake (some women prefer to apply liner first, shadow after). Pencil eyeliners, like eyebrow pencils, are about 50 percent wax. The liquid liners are about 50 percent water and contain thickeners and emulsifiers.

Work slowly and carefully when you apply eyeliner. The American Medical Association's committee concerned with skin health and cosmetics advises that if you are not pleased with the way you have applied your liner, you should either leave it alone or wash it off completely and not attempt to reapply it for several hours. Immediate reapplications are very hard on the eyes.

Lining the Lid Ledge and Other No-Nos

A common cause of eye irritation is applying the eyeliner pencil *inside* the edge of the eyelid. Use it only on the outside of the lid. It is best to keep all foreign matter out of the eye. If you use a pencil, sharpen it just before using; it will be cleaner as well as easier to use. Another important health point: Do not moisten your eye pencil with saliva or water, as this creates an environment for bacteria.

The tiny paint brushes included with liquid liner can also host bacteria. Do not keep a liquid liner more than a few months. Liquid liners generally are very drying and are difficult to blend.

If you find you have an allergic reaction to a product, the problem could be the preservative paraben. Try switching to paraben-free products such as Clinique's Basic Eye Emphasizer and Resistant Eyeliner.

Some Eyeliner Yes-Yeses

In applying eyeliner, you can echo the shape of the shadow—heavy toward the center for widely spaced eyes, heavy on the outer edges for closely spaced eyes. Whether to keep the liner's work cleanly sharp or smudged is a matter of preference, but smudging can be irritating to the skin of your eyelid. If you prefer a softer line, use a powder pencil or a soft cream pencil. Here are some popular products:

- Madeleine Mono Indian Eyes (Madeleine Mono)
- Eye Accento (Princess Marcella Borghese)
- Eye Contouring Pencil (Estée Lauder)
- Accents Crayon (L'Oréal)

When applying your liner, hold the skin to prevent it from dragging, and work from the outer corner toward the inner corner. Look down into a mirror or, if looking straight ahead, hold the lid down slightly.

Two Eyeliner Color Tips

- Use a bluish line around the eyes to make them look clearer if they are bloodshot.
- Dot a bit of pink near your nose on the inner corner of your eye if you want a lively bright look when you are not feeling great.

The Latest in Eye Makeup

Permanent eyelining, also called eye tattooing, is a new procedure usually performed by a dermatologist, ophthalmologist, or plastic surgeon. It was developed for women who for various reasons have difficulty applying eye makeup, are allergic to eye makeup, simply do not want to take the time to apply makeup, or want to look made up at all times.

Eyes are lined with black, light or dark brown, or gray dye of iron oxide and titanium oxide pigments. Once the procedure is undertaken the color *cannot* be removed or even lightened. The procedure is performed in the doctor's office with an electric needle and under local anesthesia; dye is injected into the lid in a row of close-set dots.

The biggest drawback seems to be the commitment to permanent eyeliner. Complications include temporary puffiness and bruising, discoloration of the skin at the sites of dye injection (which can appear even a few years later), loss of eyelashes (follicles can be destroyed if the technique is performed improperly), and occasional systemic reaction to the implant material or migration of the coloring material, causing a smeared effect.

Mascara

Eyelashes draw attention to your eyes. They also protect your eyes from dust and debris. Eyelashes grow slowly—it takes about three months for an eyelash to grow full length—so treat them tenderly.

Start with proper lash care. To increase the impact of their eyes, many women curl their lashes before applying mascara. If you do this, first oil your lashes with castor oil, and then apply a bit of oil to the rubber rim of the curler before you use it. (This is also the time to check the rubber rim to be sure it is in good condition and will not damage your lashes.) Tighten the curler slightly on the lashes and hold for a moment or two. Then dry your lashes carefully by blotting them on tissue before applying mascara.

Mascara Choices—What You Want from a Mascara

Most mascaras now come in liquid form and contain many colors, thickeners, and preservatives. Some products include lash builders or mascara extenders, which are usually nylon or rayon fibers. Avoid fiber builders if you wear contact lenses, because small fibers can drop under a lens and cause severe irritation; they can also bat against the plastic lenses of eyeglasses and eventually cloud or scratch the lenses.

Here are several products that include lash builders:

- Fresh Lash Mascara (Maybelline)
- Immencils Gentle Lash Thickener (Lancôme)
- Lavish Lash Building Mascara (Elizabeth Arden)

Mascara has a bad record for causing tearing, itching, and swelling of eyelids in some women. If you can't tolerate mascara, try a hypoallergenic brand and avoid switching brands, since that seems often to trigger reactions. And use mascara only on the outer tips of the lashes. Some mascaras are still mercury-based (as are some lens solutions) and can be irritating; avoid them if you can. Cake mascaras are the gentlest. Waterproof mascaras are ideal for women active in sports. However, waterproof mascaras are the most difficult to remove.

Do not keep mascara longer then six months.

How to Apply Mascara

Powder your lashes first. The best position to take to apply mascara is to lay a mirror flat on top of a table and look down into it. You will be less likely to squint. Always check your mascara wand to be sure the color is evenly distributed along it; most clogs and clumps start on the brush and are transferred to your lashes.

Apply a light coat of mascara. Powder your lashes again by closing your eyes and whisking your lashes with a soft brush. Then apply another coat of mascara. The powder helps to dry the mascara quickly, adds to the buildup, and allows you to add up to five coats of mascara without clumping.

You can avoid the most common mistake of an unwanted blob of mascara landing on your lower lid by placing a small piece of ordinary tissue under the lashes before applying your mascara. The tissue acts as a shield. On lower lashes remember to apply mascara from the inner corner to the outer corner—not up and down.

How to Reshape Your Eyes with Mascara

For daytime wear choose a black or brown mascara, depending on your coloring. For evening wear you can use almost any color; black is always effective.

Here are some illusions you can create:

- To enlarge eyes that are small, apply the thickest coat to the outer lashes.
- To offset deep-set eyes, use mascara only on the tips of your lashes. This will draw attention upward and outward.
- To deemphasize protruding or bulging eyes, use only a light coating of mascara.

Removing Mascara Without Damaging Your Lashes

Removing mascara can be as much or more of a job than applying it. Few mascaras come off with soap and water. Oily eye makeup removers are usually based on mineral oil, often with perfume added; nonoily products use boric acid and other dissolvents. Oily or saturated pads are easiest to use, but they can blur your vision for a moment because any oil that gets into the eyes is irritating. They also often leave a sooty circle around the entire eye. Leaving mascara or eye makeup on overnight will cause your skin, particularly the skin under the eyes, to dry.

For removing mascara and other eye makeup, use a product designed for this purpose or baby oil or petroleum jelly:

1. Moisten a cotton swab, cotton ball, or cotton pad and work from the base of the lash outward.
2. Keep a tissue under the lash to absorb extra oil and the color that will be washed away.
3. Do not rub. Blot.

Whatever procedure you use, always rinse your eyes well with cool tap water after removing eye makeup.

Eyebrows

Delicately arched or richly luxurious, your brows frame your face and are the perfect setting for your eyes. Brows are so much a part of our total image that some famous people can be recognized by their eyebrows alone: Who could imagine Greta Garbo with heavy brows or Brooke Shields with sparse ones?

The more natural-looking your brows are, the more they enhance your personality. Never try to reshape your brows completely—what you should strive for is making them look their best. Because they can be so arresting, you can use your eyebrows to create an illusion that affects the rest of your face. Brows can make your other features look wider, narrower, longer, or shorter—or just more interesting. Modifying the shape of your natural brows can also make your eyes look larger, more alert, and more open. The shape of your brows can even make you look older or younger.

How to Care for Your Brows

The hair of the eyebrows is like that of the lashes. Although it is short, it diverts perspiration, dust, and dirt from the sensitive eye area. As with the hair of the scalp, brows and lashes have a normal shedding cycle—the life of the hair of the eyebrows is about four or five months.

Groom your brows often: Use a small eyebrow brush or a child's very soft toothbrush to brush your brows lightly at least once a day. Brushing keeps them gleaming and in place. (When you wash your face your brows are stripped of their natural oils.) The best time for brushing is before applying eye pencil and after removing it. You can touch up eyebrows with a little bit of hair spray or mousse to keep them in shape.

If the hairs of your brows grow very long, trim them neatly with small, sharp scissors. If the hairs grow unevenly or sparsely in some areas, you can fill in by using an eyebrow pencil. As with an eyeliner pencil, sharpen the pencil directly before use to keep it pointed and clean. The shape of the brows can be enhanced and sparse spots evened by carefully stroking with the pencil to imitate actual hairs.

How to Shape Your Brows to Enhance Your Eyes

The natural arch of the eyebrows follows the bony structure of the orbit underneath. Most people have a disorderly growth of hairs both above and below the natural line. Those below can be removed with tweezers to give a well-defined look to the brows. (Those above should be brushed downward, not tweezed.) However, making eyebrows too thin can make your face look flat and eyes puffy.

Here is how to determine your best eyebrow and facial proportions:

- The highest point of the eyebrow should be directly above the outer edge of the pupil, the center of the colored portion of the eye, when you look straight ahead.
- The brow should start directly above the inner corner of the eye.
- To locate where the brow should end, imagine a line drawn diagonally from the tip of your nostril (left nostril for the left eye, right nostril for the right eye) past the outer tip of the eye and extended upward toward the temple. The point where this imaginary line hits the eyebrows should be the outer end of the brow.

How to Use Your Brows to Make Your Face Look More Symmetrical

Your brows should be symmetrical and make your eyes look more symmetrical, too. The loveliest brows (or eyes) look odd unless the right and left match each other as closely as possible.

The following principles indicate where the brows should be on an ideally proportioned face; use the information as a rough guide to making your own individual features more balanced.

- *Round face:* Arching the brows makes the face appear narrower. Start tweezing directly above the inside corner of the eye and extend the brow to the end of the cheekbone.
- *Long face:* Do not arch the brows; keep them full, heavy, and straight. Do not extend the brow past the outer edge of the eye.
- *Square face:* Arch the brows, with the height of the arch near the outer ends of the brows, over the outer corners of the eyes.
- *Low forehead:* Use a clear, high arch to give yourself height.
- *Close-set eyes:* Be sure the area between the brows is open and as wide as possible by starting the brows slightly more to the center of the eye and ending the brows closer to the temples.
- *Wide-set eyes:* Make the eyes seem closer together by starting the brows near the bridge of the nose.
- If your eyes seem to droop slightly downward on the outer edges, giving you a sad, bleary expression, raise your brows at the ends, and use shadow to fill in the area.

If one eye or brow is different from the other—smaller, shorter, tilts, etc.—use makeup to create a visual illusion of symmetry. If, on the other hand, you enjoy an odd quirk of a brow, you can enhance that to create a focus on your eyes and brow.

Tweezing—When Your Brows Overpower You

Because of the sensitivity of the skin around the eyes, you may find that tweezing your brows can be painful. You can also have the hair of the brows waxed or bleached. Do not attempt to wax or bleach your brows yourself. Dyeing, bleaching, or waxing of eyebrows should be done only by a careful, trained professional cosmetician. For permanent changes, you can have professional electrolysis.

Tweezing, like waxing, can damage hair follicles; after several years of tweezing, many women notice that in the area between the brows or in other tweezed areas the hair is sparse. Tweezing can cause redness and swelling; so do not tweeze soon before going out.

After tweezing, rinse the area carefully with cool water and apply an antiseptic. Brush the brows in place and then use an eyebrow pencil to fill in

How to Tweeze Your Brows
with a Minimum of Discomfort

For a professional-looking tweezing that should last a week or two (with touch-ups) collect the following items:

Tweezers (many styles are available; find the one you like best)
Small brush   Warm water   Cotton balls   Magnifying mirror
Antiseptic lotion   Astringent   Eye cream   Anesthetic ointment

Wash your face to rid your skin of any eye makeup; rinse with warm water. Soak the cotton balls in warm water and apply them to your eyebrows so that the skin and brows are softened.

Most of the shaping should be done from the underbrow. Brush the hairs upward and shape the lower section, working in the direction in which the hair grows. If it is very painful, you can apply an anesthetic ointment (e.g. Xylocaine 2.5% ointment, manufactured by Astra) to this area. Hold the skin so you are not pulling it more than necessary.

1. Start by removing the hairs between the brows. Stretch the skin very slightly or keep it taut with your index and middle fingers of your free hand.
2. Grasp each hair individually with the tweezers, and pull it quickly in the direction in which it grows. Tweeze the hairs between the brows first.
3. To camouflage the few ragged hairs from above the brow line, brush them downward. Do not tweeze.
4. Most important, work slowly and don't overtweeze. Remember, it takes about five months for new brow hair to restore an over-tweezed clump.

thin areas or to create the effect you want. When using a pencil, never draw one long, harsh line. For a natural look, use short strokes in the direction of hair growth.

Eyebrow pencils and eyeliner pencils are interchangeable most of the time. Some eyeliner pencils are softer and waxier—more smudgeable—than the brow pencils, but the formulas are similar. In reshaping or filling in the brows when the arch is too high, lower it by thickening the brow under the arch; when the arch is too low, raise it by adding a few pencil strokes to the top of the arch.

Many women have coarse and resistant brows, and others find that with age their brows get more bristly. To keep them neat and to keep the color smooth and even if your brows are graying, you can coat them with a thin cover of mascara in medium or dark brown (black seems too harsh for all but the youngest brunettes). The waxy mascara keeps the brows neat indefinitely.

Keep tweezers and brushes clean and as close to bacteria-free as possible by wiping your tweezers with alcohol both before and after use. Clean your brush by whisking it through alcohol also. (For more on removing unwanted hair, see chapter 22.)

Eyebrow and Eyelash Dyeing

If you want your lashes or brows bleached or tinted, have the work done professionally. If you color your hair, your hairdresser can lighten brows at the same time. Ask about the dye that will be used, and do not permit aniline or coal-tar dyes to be used on your lashes. Dye of whatever kind should be used only on the lashes themselves; the skin of the eyes and eye area should be protected with a thick coating of petroleum jelly and paper shields. (For more about eyes—how to make them fresh and attractive and how to deal with puffy eyes—see chapter 20.)

Eyeglasses and Sunglasses

Glasses give you an extra opportunity to enhance your best facial features and draw attention away from those that are less than perfect. Glasses come in an endless variety of shapes, colors, styles, and materials. The lenses, frames, and earpieces change with the tides of fashion, but within the context of any particular fashion a few basics always apply when you reach the point of selecting the color, weight, and shape that is best for you.

Most metal frames are made from alloys that contain nickel, an allergen that affects many women. If you are allergic to nickel, avoid metal frames. If your nose is oily, the pressure of the nose rest against your skin can lead to acne mechanica. Select the lightest-weight frames possible.

Eyeglasses for everyday wear are usually clear glass. (Glass lenses transmit only UVA rays, while plastic lenses transmit UVA and UVB rays.) For sunglasses most experts recommend neutral-colored lenses—gray, smoke, or gray-green. Darker green and gray lenses protect more effectively than pink or yellow. Surprisingly, very dark lenses are not always effective in protecting your eyes.

Sunglasses reduce squinting (which contributes to the formation of fine lines), protect against glare, guard against dust, and reduce the chance of the skin around your eyes darkening. Wear them at the beach, in the desert, or for water sports.

Even if you wear contact lenses, it is wise to wear regular sunglasses in windy weather to protect your eyes from the drying effects of the air passing over your face and causing eyes to tear, burn, and itch. (Never rub your eyelids; doing so will irritate the thin skin.)

Sunglasses also guard against sunburned corneas. It is now thought there is a link between ultraviolet rays and the development of cataracts. Prescription lenses that block all ultraviolet light are available for those with light-sensitive eyes. UV 400, Univis, and Contrast Control are among the photoprotective lenses available.

When you wear sunglasses, you can further protect the delicate skin around your eyes with a thick coating of sunscreen designed for the eye area.

If You Wear Glasses

Here are some tips that may help you integrate glasses into a beautiful image and an active life:

- If you are farsighted (you need glasses for reading but not at the movies), remember that your lenses will magnify your eyes for anyone looking at you, so your eye makeup should be soft and subdued.
- If you are nearsighted (you need glasses for long-distance vision), wear strong, even dramatic eye colorings or your eyes will be lost behind your corrective lenses.
- If you are active in sports or other vigorous pursuits, consider sports glasses with stronger frames and special nose and ear pads to minimize rubbing, a good investment in beauty. The lenses are shatterproof and resist scratches.
- For wear in the sun, water sports, or winter sports such as skiing, look for a wraparound style of sunglasses. Much of the irritating glare that causes squinting comes in at the corners of the eyes.
- For swimming, select leakproof goggles that cover as much of your face as possible. They will be more comfortable and less pressuring than the small round cups used by many swimmers. Use petroleum jelly applied to the rubber seal to help keep water out.

A Word About Contact Lenses

If you are a contact lens wearer, insert lenses before applying makeup, and take out lenses before attempting to remove makeup. Avoid lash builders, waterproof mascaras, and glittery shadows, which can flake.

11

FOR KISSES
SWEETER THAN . . .

Fashion magazines are full of pretty lips—soft, moist, and pouty—often announcing a lipstick that can turn dull to dazzling. Millions are spent on lipsticks each year. Pretty lips can be your best feature—if you know how to cater to the special needs of your lips' special skin. (I find a lipstick is the fastest way to change my look, and my outlook.)

Lips are different from skin on other parts of the body in three ways:

1. Lips are composed of mucous membranelike tissue and have no horny epidermal layer to protect them.
2. Lips do not have oil glands to provide natural oils as a defense against the evaporation of moisture.
3. Lips do not produce melanin, the protective color that is in skin.

Without these three skin defenses, lips are very vulnerable. Yet they are also amazingly resilient. And a lavish supply of sense receptors lets them detect the most delicate touch. They are perfect as an erotic organ.

Lovely lips have several enemies to beware of.

Exposure. Lips that are dry, chapped, and peeling defy cosmetic coverage and are prone to infection as well. Since they are constantly exposed to the elements—sun, wind, and cold—dry lips are victim to many of the same problems that affect the skin. In addition, they are exposed to potential irritants in food, cosmetics, cigarettes, and any foreign substance your fingers may carry to them.

Allergies. Once the thin, delicate covering of the lips is cracked, other problems may follow: infections that can cause swelling and blistering. Allergic reactions to cosmetics, balms, mentholated products, and even toothpastes and mouthwashes are not uncommon. Luckily, restoring injured lips to good health is relatively easy. Because a rich blood supply is available to them, they heal quickly.

Habits. Lips may be damaged and aged by excessive use—for example, by constantly sucking on cigarettes, gesturing, pulling at the lips, licking them, and other harmful habits. Avoid exercises that stretch, pull, and abuse the lips' muscle tissue and become aware of any habits you might have that could damage the skin on or around your lips. Laugh . . . but do not grimace.

Teeth. Since lips rest against the teeth, good dental hygiene is vital to lip care. Without the backing of strong gums and teeth, your lips, no matter how healthy, recede unattractively into the cavity of your mouth. To avoid aging lips, frequent visits to the dentist are a must.

Summer Lips

Sun has a profound effect on all skin. Because they lack melanin, your body's natural color sunscreen, and have no protective outer layer of horny skin cells, your lips are almost defenseless. Furthermore, the saliva that constantly bathes your lips' surface actually concentrates the sun's ultraviolet rays, making your lips burn even more quickly. Years of exposure to the sun can cause actinic cheilitis, discussed later in this chapter.

Since your lips cannot protect themselves, lip balms and lipsticks are more than cosmetic; they are essential protection against the effects of sun, wind, and cold. They prevent drying and chapping and even help protect against cancer of the lips. Two to try are Presun 15 Ultra Sunscreen Lip Protector (Westwood) and Bain de Soleil Ultra Sunblock Lip Balm (Charles of the Ritz).

Lipstick Bonus

The best all-around help for sun-threatened lips is to wear lipstick that includes a sunscreen in its formula. The sunscreen will absorb or block out the sun's ultraviolet rays, and the pigments and colors in the lipstick will further help to protect against the sun's penetration.

One of every eight to ten women is allergic to the common sunscreen ingredient PABA. If you are one of them, switch to PABA-free lip products such as:

• Sun Stick (Cooper Labs)
• Piz Buin Stick (Greiter)
• TiScreen Lip and Face Protectant (T/I Pharmaceuticals)

If you prefer a natural look for beach and sports activities, use a neutral, skin-color lipstick or cover stick. Forget the gloss that comes with most lipsticks, as it merely focuses the sun's rays on your lips, very much the way a lens is sometimes used by campers to focus light on a bit of paper to start a fire. For maximum protection against the sun use a thick, densely colored lipstick, and try to find a matte finish, as frosted lipsticks focus light almost as much as glosses.

Nine Lip Tips for Smooth Summers

1. Choose lip products that contain a sunscreen.
2. Add a layer of lip sunscreen (preferably with an SPF of 15) under or over your lipstick (even better, under *and* over).
3. Select lip products that will not be easily washed away by saliva.
4. Always keep some sort of barrier between your lips and the drying, burning outside world.
5. Apply sunscreen to your lips a half hour before sun exposure.
6. Reapply sunscreen often—after swimming, eating, or drinking or after a few hours of wear.
7. Do not substitute sunscreen lotions or other products made for face and body skin. They will not work as well as specially formulated lip preparations and may even cause problems.
8. Do not use any product that includes alcohol, as it may cause drying and stinging of the lip surface.
9. For maximum protection on the beach, in the water, and on the ski slopes, use total sunblock such as zinc oxide paste.

Water Sports Protection

If you participate in water sports, it is imperative that you protect your lips with emollient sunscreen products that are formulated to stay on your lips in spite of splashes and spray. Petroleum jelly is a poor choice because it acts as a gloss and focuses the sun's rays on your lips. When you sail or swim, the upper lip becomes as vulnerable to sun damage as the lower lip usually is, because the sun is reflected upward from the water. (Landlubbers, especially in cities, are not immune to upper-lip sun damage. Concrete pavements reflect light very much the way water does. Your upper lip and the area under your chin can become sunburned from that reflection, just as they can from sun reflected off the water.)

Help for Sunburned Lips

If your lips have been sunburned, cool compresses of equal parts of water and milk can help ease the irritation and pain. You can also use an anesthetic ointment such as Xylocaine 2.5% (Astra) or any nonprescription steroid ointment two or three times a day. These over-the-counter preparations will help ease the discomfort of burned lips.

You can wear lipstick over sunburned lips. First apply a medicated balm, then use a creamy but nonglossy lipstick, and stay out of the sun. Avoid preparations containing benzocaine, a primary cause of allergic reactions.

Other Sun-Related Lip Problems

Reactions to Food

Lips react to photosensitizers just as skin does. The following foods and spices have photosensitizing properties when in contact with the lips:

Celery	Bitter orange	Carrots
Dill	Parsnips	Cinnamon
Figs	Lime	Lemon

The possibility of anyone rubbing parsnips on her skin may seem remote, but when you eat, you do just that to your lips. Gin and tonics and other drinks containing lime, vegetable juices, lemonades, and foods seasoned with cinnamon, such as Danish pastries, are summer favorites. Remember their photosensitizing ability if you are planning to be in the sun.

Reactions to Medicines and Chemicals

While most lipsticks serve to protect your lips, others may actually do more harm than good. Lipsticks containing dyes made from certain tar derivatives can cause a photosensitizing reaction, actually increasing your chances for sunburn and cracked lips. Check the labels on your lipstick and avoid eosin if your lips react to the sun. So-called indelible dyes such as bromofluorescin are also photosensitizing. Fragrances used in lipsticks can cause an allergic reaction resembling dry, chapped lips.

Medications that can react with sunlight include:

- Tetracycline and related antibiotics, often prescribed in the treatment of acne
- Thiazides, sometimes used by those who need a diuretic
- Phenothiazines, used in psychiatric therapy

These may lead to summertime sunburning of the lips because of increased sensitivity. If you are taking these medications, stay out of the sun. (For more about sun-reactive foods and medications, see chapter 6.)

Winter Lips

Winter is the season for dry, chapped lips. Cold dry air that is heated for comfort in your home or office becomes drier still, so lips tend to become dry and chapped from both outdoor winter cold and indoor winter heat.

Large buildings—offices, department stores, hospitals, airline terminals (and planes), and hotels—tend to be exceptionally dry in the wintertime. Patients entering hospitals and persons taking trips usually notice dry lips almost from the outset. Blistex (Blistex), a lip ointment, is used by NASA crews on space shuttle flights as a guard against dry, parched lips. Here on Earth you can also use petroleum jelly, Vaseline Constant Care Lip Balm (Chesebrough-Pond's), Carmex (Carma), or Eight Hour Cream Lipcare Stick (Elizabeth Arden).

The Dry/Lick Cycle

When the air is very dry, it dries your lips and you tend to lick them to remoisten them. The more you lick, the drier your lips actually become. The moisture you put on your lips evaporates very rapidly, and the constant moistening and evaporation causes chapping, just as frequent wetting and drying result in dry skin.

Common colds, so prevalent every winter, add to lip dryness as well. When you have a fever with your cold you often breathe faster, or hyperventilate. A congested nose makes you breathe through your mouth; increased salivation chaps lips further. In addition, many over-the-counter cold and cough drugs include antihistamines, and dry mouth and dry lips are common side effects of these drugs. Other medications that dry lips are decongestants, diuretics, anticholinergics, and Accutane. Other lip chappers: dental malocclusion and constant chewing of gum or hard candy.

Winter Sports

Winter sports can play havoc with your lips. The clear, dry mountain air, bright sun, and snow-reflected glare at ski resorts make sunscreen lip protection as important to winter visitors as to summer athletes at the beach. As in the summer, wear a lipstick with a sunscreen all day long; use a *lip block* on the ski slopes.

Much winter sports equipment is made of metal—be careful not to touch skin or lips to them in cold weather. You risk tissue freezing to the metal and then tearing when you pull away.

Help for Winter Lips

Humidifying the air of your home and office will help prevent wintertime dry lips and skin. Besides treating the air surrounding you, you can help your lips directly:

- Apply a lip balm to your lips every night before retiring.If you find your lips very dry, keep them covered with lip balm at all times.
- Drink additional fluids—several ounces of water every few hours. With age, the ability of the skin's cells to retain moisture decreases, so each new winter the dryness of your body may seem to increase.
- Use lipsticks with built-in moisturizers. Lip Smoothers Plus (Merle Norman), Lip Treatment Moisturizer (Borghese), and Longline Lip Polisher (Estée Lauder) are three good possibilities.

Cheilitis

A persistent inflammation of one or both lips just at the point where the lip skin meets the normal skin (the vermilion border) is called cheilitis. It occurs in every age group and both sexes. If it is brought on by exposure to the sun it is called actinic cheilitis, which is associated with dry, scaly, chapped lips. Cosmetics and a host of other products can also be suspect.

Cheilitis from lipsticks usually appears a week or more after a new type of lipstick is used. It may also suddenly develop from a lipstick that has been used without problems for weeks or months. It usually appears as dryness and fissuring on the lips, particularly at the vermilion border; the corners of the mouth are seldom involved. The severity of lipstick cheilitis varies from a mild redness, scaling, and fissuring to a swollen and crusting condition that is quite unpleasant.

Contact or Allergic Cheilitis

Considering how many millions of Americans use lipstick, the rareness of cosmetic cheilitis is remarkable. One explanation for the good record of the cosmetics industry is that all cosmetics must be carefully tested and screened to receive the approval of the Food and Drug Administration (FDA). However, some cases do occur. It is possible to use a product safely without any problem for weeks or months and then suddenly and unpredictably find that you are allergic to it. Certain dyes, fragrances, or flavoring agents used to make lipstick taste pleasant are most likely to be the cause of an allergic reaction.

If you suffer allergic reactions to foods or other substances, the chances are above average that sooner or later you will have an allergic reaction to some cosmetics products. Here is a list of ingredients found in various popular lipsticks that have been associated with allergies:

Castor oil	Lanolin	Antioxidant	Cinnamon
Beeswax	D&C dyes	Alcohol	Cocoa butter
Carnauba wax	Perfumes	Oleyl carmine dye	

If you are allergic to cinnamon, which is in cosmetics as well as food, you probably will also have a reaction to other products (including balsam of Peru) used in perfumes and in dentistry in some liquid cements. Glossy lipsticks with high concentrations of lanolin are more associated with allergic reactions than other styles are. The following foods can also be offenders when in contact with the lips: oranges, lemons, artichokes, mangoes, carrots, and coffee.

Lip pencils used to draw color lines along the vermilion border are another possible source of trouble. Such pencils are intensively loaded with pigments.

Women with sensitivity to nickel can suffer lip irritations as the result of contact with metallic lipstick containers or nickel-plated objects such as coins, keys, pins, paper clips, or bobby pins held between their lips. Some women are allergic to nail polish; if they touch their lips with nails still wet with polish, they can develop allergy-triggered lip problems. (Sensitivity to nail polish is usually a reaction to toluene sulfonamide formaldehyde resin. Hypoallergenic polishes usually contain an alkaloid resin instead.)

If you have an allergic reaction, the first step to take is to stop using any product you think might have caused it. If you manage to identify the culprit, study the list of ingredients on its label and compare the labels of your other cosmetics. By a process of elimination, you may be able to identify the problem ingredient and so avoid using products with that ingredient in the future. Keep trying new products until you find one that works for you. If your investigations are getting nowhere, your dermatologist may be able to perform patch tests to determine the exact ingredient that is troubling you.

Treatment for Allergic Cheilitis

The way to treat allergic cheilitis is to first find and get rid of the substance containing the allergen. Then follow the appropriate guidelines for relief of symptoms and to promote healing.

- For swelling of the lips, apply compresses soaked in ice-cold water at least twice a day.
- When swelling of the lips is accompanied by cracking and crusting, you can use an over-the-counter preparation, either Bacitracin (Fougera) or Polysporin Ointment (Burroughs Wellcome). These are less sensitizing than some other antibiotic preparations.
- When the entire mouth is swollen, sucking on small pieces of ice may be helpful.
- For general lip relief, you can also visit your local veterinary supply store. Bag Balm, an ointment used for animals' udders, is an excellent balm for humans, too. It is also sold in some health food stores. (Check with your physician if you are a nursing mother; this might work well for nipple irritations, too.)

Perlèche

Lip tissue can mirror faulty nutrition. Angular cheilitis or perlèche—a French term, pronounced "pair-lesh"—refers to a condition marked by cracks at the corners of the mouth. The disorder is most common in older people who wear dentures or are missing teeth. Rough handling when using dental floss can also be a cause. Perlèche may indicate a deficiency of riboflavin (vitamin B₂). Eating foods high in riboflavin—milk, yogurt, oatmeal, spinach, broccoli, and liver—helps eradicate this problem. In addition to vitamin B₂ deficiency, vitamin B₆, protein, and iron deficiencies have been implicated as possible causes of cracks at the corners of the mouth. (On the other hand, an excess of vitamins A and E can cause chapped lips.)

Other possible causes of the condition include bacterial infections and thrush, a yeast infection of the mouth. Any kind of persistent lip chapping will create a yeast-inviting situation.

Some people are predisposed to perléche because of grooves at the corners of the mouth. Collagen injections can fill out these grooves. Perlèche usually responds well to an over-the-counter cream, Micatin (Ortho Pharmaceutical), used three times a day in conjunction with Bacitracin (Fougera), an over-the-counter ointment. The latter works wonders when rubbed on the inflamed skin surrounding your lips.

Lip Cancer

Because lips lack a protective coat and color, they are very susceptible to cancer, particularly squamous cell carcinoma. Lip cancer is rare in women who regularly use lipstick (because of the extra protection) but relatively common in men. Smoking may also contribute to lip cancer.

Ultraviolet radiation from the sun appears to be the greatest source of trouble. The lower lip is most at risk to damage from the sun's rays because of its position, so always keep your lower lip coated. Clouds are no protection against the sun's direct rays. No matter what the weather, be sure to use protection every summer day from 10 A.M. to after 2 P.M. in northern latitudes and all day long on a Caribbean or Mexican vacation.

If your lips have a nonhealing crack or sore or develop a growth that resembles a wart, see your dermatologist immediately.

Herpes Simplex of the Lips (Herpes Labialis)

The common cold sore or fever blister, which many people are surprised to learn is a viral infection caused by the herpes simplex virus, afflicts so many that it is second only to the common cold in prevalence. Herpes simplex of the lips can be brought on by stress, exposure to sun or wind, pregnancy, menstruation, illness accompanied by fever, a cold, or physical trauma. After an initial attack, the virus becomes latent, staying in your system. It can remain latent for life or it can reemerge, usually as a result of one of these triggers.

Tingling and itching usually precede the onset of a cold sore. The affected area first reddens, then swells into a blister that breaks after a few days and forms a honey-colored crust. The sores begin to heal within four days to two weeks, then disappear.

Herpes is highly contagious; you can easily infect other parts of your body as well as other people after a blister has appeared. However, the presence of herpes simplex of the lips does not necessarily indicate sexual transmission or the presence of genital herpes.

To avoid contracting the virus, do not use lipstick testers directly on the lips (use the wrist) or share drinking glasses, eating utensils, etc. People with a history of cold sores should avoid sun and wind exposure as well as any irritation of the lips. Use sun-blocking lip balms and lipsticks with sun-screens added. If a sore is present, be careful when drying your face so as not to spread the infection to other areas, especially the eyes.

If a cold sore appears, applying ice cubes will reduce the swelling. Anesthetic over-the-counter ointments such as Blistex Medicated Lip Ointment (Blistex), Carmex (Carma), or Xylocaine 2.5% ointment (Astra) offer topical relief from the discomfort. Acyclovir (trade name Zovirax) is the most effective antiviral agent in the treatment of herpes simplex. Available in the form of Zovirax ointment and pills (from Burroughs-Wellcome) by prescription only, it suppresses the virus in infected areas without affecting healthy cells. Zovirax also relieves the symptoms, speeds healing, and shortens the duration of the infection and the contagious period. Though it does not eradicate the latent form of the virus, this medication can help prevent recurrences in many cases if used during the first attack.

You can use lipstick over a cold sore, but direct application will probably be uncomfortable. Apply an ointment or lip balm first, then use a softer moisturizing lipstick such as Lip Smoothers Plus, Lip Treatment Moisturizer, and Longline Lip Polisher.

Wrinkled Skin Above the Lips

Many women ask why men's lips do not seem to age as quickly as women's do. Men seldom have "prune lips," the bane of many women. The skin above and below men's lips is thicker and is reinforced from within by numerous mustache and beard hairs embedded in it, so it does not wrinkle as quickly. Thus supported, lips retain their fullness. Women who use wax to remove the hair on their upper lip deprive the lip of the support of these hairs and are more vulnerable to wrinkles than women who do not.

Warding Off the "Older Mouth"

As we age, the collagen and elastin in our skin ages and changes; our skin becomes weaker and less elastic. A similar process occurs, much more rapidly, when we allow the sun to beat down on unprotected lips. We get dry, wrinkled lips and fine lines around the mouth. (Smoking accelerates this process.) Facial lines around the mouth become even more conspicuous when lipstick bleeds, drawing lip color off the lip and into the tiny creases, feathering the edge of your lipstick. (How to avoid this problem is described in "Applying Lip Color," later in this chapter.)

Aging lips can also develop spots similar to skin "liver spots" and broken capillaries.

A look of age can be accented by failure to moisturize the area, which is often very dry. Although dryness does not in itself cause wrinkles, it makes them more obvious. Remember to apply a moisturizer with sunscreen to this area. Surprisingly, this area is often forgotten when moisturizer is applied to the face. Using a moisturizer here consistently is essential.

A Plan of Action

Start with the lips themselves. Lip-smoothing creams and special ointments designed to be used as under-lipstick creams have recently become very popular. Most of them work well because they act as barriers to evaporation of the moisture on the lips' surface; they also are thickly pigmented and actually fill in tiny cracks and fissures in the tissue at the very edge of the lip.

Next, turn to the task of erasing or camouflaging wrinkling *above* the lips. Several modes of treatment are available.

Temporary

• First bombard the area above the upper lip with moisturizers.
• Long-term usage of Retin-A preparations can be beneficial.
• Apply one of the new fix-your-lips preparations to coat the lips themselves. This will cause a slight swelling in the skin above the lip, which will plump out or fill the furrows you see as lines. (I like Visible Difference Lip-Fix Creme from Elizabeth Arden.)
• Use a lip pencil to outline the lips at the vermilion border. This will hold the lip color in place. If this is difficult, use lip pencils to coat the entire lip.

Permanent or Semipermanent

Collagen injections can be used to remedy deep lines. They work by pumping up from under the surface of the skin. The effects of the procedure frequently last up to one year before touch-up treatments are needed. Collagen injected directly into the vermilion border can make lips fuller and more defined.

Dermabrasion and chemical peeling are also used to combat lip wrinkles. These procedures involve abrading or peeling away the tiny lines of the upper lips. Some doctors prefer dermabrasion for skin that is not sun-damaged and chemical peeling for skin that is. Both procedures leave the skin pink and vulnerable for weeks or even months. To protect it from the sun you will need to wear a sunblock on your upper lip (which you should do anyway). Fall is the best time for both procedures, because the sunlight is not as strong and the cold, chapping winds of winter have not yet begun.

Lip Cosmetics—The Choices

Women have not always worn lip cosmetics. Historians trace today's customs back to the brilliant makeup used by dancers in the 1910 Paris performances of the Russian Ballet, but only when Theda Bara, an exotic star of the silent screen, popularized lipstick several years later was it considered a cosmetic for everyone. Lipstick is still the most important lip cosmetic; pencils and crayons are simply lipstick with more wax and more pigments in their formulas.

Lip gloss is a relatively new makeup product. Its ingredients are quite similar to those in lipstick, but it usually has a higher percentage of oil or petroleum jelly, which gives the lips a light, natural, finished look. Unfortunately, many women apply lip gloss by rubbing the surface of their lips with their fingers, transferring dirt and oils from their fingers to their lips. A better idea is to use a lip brush for the application of both lipstick and gloss.

Applying Lip Color

Lips are the easiest of your features to alter, and if you change your mind, all you need to do is remove the lipstick and start again. You can paint on almost any expression you want with a strongly colored lipstick, but the effect may look clownlike unless you very carefully blend the edges.

The following sequence will help you keep your lip color on hours longer and let you remain bright-lipped and unfeathered while eating or drinking almost anything except very acidic or greasy foods.

1. Coat your lips with a lip ointment or an oily cream for about ten minutes before applying lip color. (Most moisturizers are not really oily enough, but a moisturizer is better than nothing.) Wipe away the oily cream using absorbent cotton saturated in warm water and a cleansing emulsion; use a downward motion on the upper lip. Work from the outer edges inward, toward the mouth (the same way that you should remove your lipstick).
2. Apply foundation to the lips to blank out as much natural color as possible, but do not make the foundation so thick that it cakes.
3. Blot well with loose translucent powder.
4. Using a lip pencil, outline the edges of your lips just beneath or above the normal surrounding skin. This is merely to define their shape. Be sure that your lip pencil is not dramatically different in color from your lipstick, or you will end up with a coloring-book mouth.
5. With a lip brush or a narrow pencil-shaped lipstick, fill with color the spaces defined by your outlines. A brush will give you the best control and make it easier to blend colors if you use more than one.

The lip color you select will have a vivid effect on your appearance and can optically change the apparent size and shape of your lips. Choose a color that coordinates with the colors of your skin, your hair, and the clothes you intend to wear. Whatever color you select, work with at least two shades so that you can control the illusion of your lips' size and fullness.

What Is the Best Color?

The names assigned to lipstick colors change with dazzling rapidity. I am constantly settling for a similar color to one I have been using because the one I want is "no longer made." This month's "shocking pink" may reemerge next month as "passion pink," enabling the lipstick behind the label to enjoy a new life with a new marketing strategy. Lipstick ingredients themselves change less often, but a few differences are worth noting.

Regular, frosted, medicated, and shimmering lipsticks are all mixtures of oil and wax in stick form with a red staining dye. Most lipstick colors are mixtures of natural pigments, synthetic coal-tar colors, and/or halogenated fluorescent derivatives that stain the lips and give the lipstick permanence or indelibility. The more indelible dyes have the potential to provoke photosensitive reactions when the lips are exposed to sunlight, increasing the wearer's risk of sunburn and dry lips and perhaps promoting irritation of the lips enough to cause the thin covering membrane to crack and peel.

To select a lipstick color that is right for you, you must evaluate your skin, hair, eyes, and wardrobe—as well as the season of the year and the effect you want to project. Sunlight reveals colors in their truest form; in the evening, electric lightbulbs may turn some colors yellowish. The bluish flourescent lights used in many offices will darken your lip color and make your skin seem pale, so use a rosy lipstick shade if you work under fluorescent light.

Try to select a lipstick color that also reflects favorably on your teeth and gums. Teeth appear whiter when contrasted with a clear, true medium red or a bluish red tone. Here are some other tips:

- If you have bluish teeth, often brought on by silver filling showing through a tooth's enamel, avoid any lipstick with a blue cast.
- If you have yellowish or pinkish teeth, avoid lipsticks with yellow or pinkish tones. (The principle is to steer clear of colors that pick up or repeat the hue you wish to avoid.)
- Pale gums look whitish and sick when in contrast with very deep shades of lipstick. If your gums are prominent, keep your lip color subdued.

D&C (Drug and Cosmetic) Colors

Among lipstick dyes in use today are D&C red colors and insoluble dyes known as lakes. Usually the darker colors last the longest. The most long-lasting of all include staining colors known as halogenated fluoresceins, which have been certified by the FDA. The staining colors are:

- D&C #5, which leaves an orange stain
- D&C #21, which leaves a medium red stain
- D&C #27, which leaves a blue-red stain

Colors to be avoided are D&C Red #9 and D&C Red #19, which have been shown to be possibly carcinogenic to laboratory animals.

Matching Your Face Shape and Size to Your Lip Shape and Size

To add beauty and character to your lips, they must be considered in the context of the shape of your entire face.

- A large face needs a mouth that is generous in proportions.
- Be careful that a round face is not echoed in rounded lips.
- A strong mouth can make your nose look shorter and smaller. If your lips are painted an intense color, attention is drawn away from your nose.
- If your jaw is narrow, small, or delicate, avoid a wide mouth that can seem to cut across your lower face.
- The ideal width of the lips is determined by the space between the pupils of the eyes; the measurements should be the same.
- For perfectly symmetrical lips the highest part of the curve of the upper lip should be directly under the center of the nostril. (You can point this top edge gently, or you can keep it as a soft curve; for most women a curved line seems more flattering.)

Adjusting the Shape and Size of Your Lips for Perfection

These are the four basic ways to change the illusion of lip size:

- *To underplay full lips:* Use lip liner just inside the natural lip line; use only soft, medium shades; avoid bright colors, frosts, and glosses. High-gloss lipsticks tend to call attention to a very full mouth.
- *To strengthen thin lips:* Use a lip pencil that is a shade darker than your lipstick along the outside of the natural lip line. Use a light but deep or dramatic shade of lipstick and a glossy finish.
- *To balance unequal lips:* If your lips are uneven in size or shape, emphasize the smaller lip by making it darker. Glossing the smaller lip also draws attention to it and makes it seem bigger.
- *To counter drooping lips:* If the outer edges of your lips droop slightly, you can achieve a youthful upward tilt by using a lip liner pencil to build up the outer corners of the upper lip very slightly.

When Your Lipstick Needs a Touch-up

For a touch-up of your lipstick, never apply a second coat of lipstick over a worn-out coat. Remove the old layer first. The temptation to touch up lipstick is strong after eating. Unfortunately, stale lipstick filled with grease from food and other foreign matter such as lint from a napkin prevents fresh color from adhering properly. Cleaning your lips by wetting them with saliva before applying color is no solution either— saliva shields the surface of your lips from the oily lipstick, so your color will vanish before very long.

If you need to touch up your lips after eating, leave the table and take a few minutes to do it right. Most people infinitely prefer lingering briefly over coffee to watching a woman pull out a lipstick at the table right after eating.

Staying Power in Lipsticks

All lipsticks contain oils, waxes, and colorants. Long-lasting lipsticks contain, in addition to the pigments or colors found in ordinary lipsticks, specific colorants called bromo acids, which have staining qualities. According to Margaret Marrison, author of a FDA pamphlet entitled *Cosmetics: Substances Beneath the Form,* many of the lipsticks popular in the 1940s and 1950s were high-stain, based on pigments no longer commonly used and apparently endowed with more holding power than today's lipsticks. Modern lipsticks are safer and the dyes are more refined. Most women, anxious to avoid what they consider a hard or obvious look in lipstick, choose not to use some colors that would actually stay on longer.

Long-lasting lipstick brands include:

- Sheer to Stay (Coty)
- L'Artiste Enduring Lipstick (L'Oréal)
- Maquiriche Lasting Mat Lip Color (Lancôme)
- Eterna "27" Enriched All-Day Lipstick (Revlon)
- Color Fast (Max Factor)
- Lip-Creme (Elizabeth Arden)
- Hours Longer (Flame Glo)
- Re-nutriv All Day Lipstick (Estée Lauder)

The lipsticks below are not labeled as long-lasting but rate high on staying power:

- Ultima II Lipstick/Pencil (Revlon)
- Lipstick (Diane von Furstenberg)

- Rouge à Lèvres (Chanel)
- Moisture Silk Lipcolor (Frances Denney)
- Moisturized Lipstick (Cover Girl)

Liquid lipsticks are brought out by cosmetics manufacturers from time to time. These products, which generally use small sponges to carry the lip color to the lips, almost never work well. They are either too runny and glossy or too drying because they contain alcohol, and they are not long-lasting.

To Fight Feathering—and Win

The following are a few products that have been developed specifically to treat problems of feathering, vanishing, and changing colors:

- Recette Merveilleuse Toure de Lèvres (Stendhal), a cream that prevents lipstick from running, even in hot weather
- B-21 (Orlane), a cream that minimizes age lines
- Lip Renew (Max Factor), a conditioning primer that controls lipstick bleeding
- Visible Difference Lip-Fix Creme (Elizabeth Arden), a colorless light cream applied under lipstick to lock it in place
- True Tone Lip Foundation Stick (Avon) for an even tone under lip color

---

Lipstick Changes as a Practical Matter

While most women are probably quite ready to acknowledge that lipstick should be chosen daily to suit the climate and their clothing, statistics show that few of us actually change our lipstick at all. Once we buy one—whether for $1.50 or $14.50—we keep on using it, unless the color changes or an allergy results.

What are the implications of the lengthy use of a single stick?

Lipsticks, like all cosmetics, do deteriorate in contact with the air and heat. If any cosmetic is exposed to much sun or remains open to the air for more than six months, the oils in it will change substantially. Such changes are most noticeable in perfumes, but lipsticks suffer, too. The shelf life of your lipsticks will depend largely on the care with which you store them; keep them sealed, cool, and protected from the direct rays of the sun. It does not hurt to replace your lipstick every six months.

12

THE BEAUTY PLUSES
AND PENALTIES OF
EXERCISE

$$L$$ike nearly everyone, I feel some concern about physical fitness. And I am one of millions who are doing something about it—jogging, jumping, and lifting to get into good shape. Exercise affects your total well-being and can change your life. It:

- Increases muscle strength and endurance
- Promotes flexibility in joints
- Is essential for bone maintenance
- Dissipates stress
- Provides an escape from pressures of work and relationships
- Aids in weight control

However, exercise may be hard on the skin. It can make you vulnerable to fungal infections, calluses, blisters, and a variety of exotic annoyances such as swimmer's itch or "bikini bottom." This chapter will help you sportsproof your skin so that you can avoid skin damage as you benefit from exercise.

The Pluses of Athletic Skin

Although no scientific data has yet been compiled to prove conclusively that exercise benefits skin health, sedentary people commonly have fragile, thin skin, while those who exercise regularly seem to have stronger, more resilient skin. By bringing more blood and oxygen to the skin for a better exchange of nutrients, exercise causes skin to grow faster and certainly appears to improve overall skin quality. In a study of exercisers and nonexercisers matched by age and skin type, researchers in Finland found that compared with those in the nonexercising control group, exercisers had:

- Greater cell-renewal capabilities
- More collagen production and therefore a denser dermis
- Better moisture retention
- More elastic (more resilient) skin
- Fewer wrinkles

Alas, they also found that the benefits of exercise ended when the exercise stopped, and that exercise in the sun does more harm than good because of the sun's aging effects.

Skin that grows faster is thicker. Why is fast-growing, thicker skin better than skin as fine and pale as exquisite parchment? For the same reasons that clothing looks fresher if you change it often and that a padded ski suit is more protection than an unpadded one. Faster means newer, fresher, and more elastic; thicker means smoother and more protective. Thick skin provides better defense against heat, cold and bruises and prevents loss of your own essential body fluids.

Exercise makes the heart work harder and sends an increased volume of blood and oxygen to the muscles and skin. Approximately 800,000 inches of blood vessels are engorged with blood during exercise, with two basic effects:

1. The level of oxygen in the blood and skin increases.
2. The temperature on the surface of the skin rises.

Higher levels of oxygen in the blood may account for the fact that many people feel refreshed and clear-headed after exercising. The greater warmth brought to the surface of the skin by increased blood circulation is beneficial in several ways. (Activity, especially if strenuous and continued for some time, tends to raise the temperature of the surface of the skin very slightly— from about 88°F when you are at rest or asleep in a moderate climate to about 93°F or higher after a workout.) It increases skin nutrition, leading to greater collagen production and thicker skin. We know that nails and hair grow faster in warm weather and the same appears to be true when skin is warmed by exercise.

Sun Sports and Sun Protection

If you exercise outdoors, remember to protect your skin from the sun. Limit outdoor sports during the late spring and summer months to shaded areas when possible, and apply a sunscreen once or twice a day at least fifteen minutes before exercising in the direct sun. (For more about the sun and sunscreens, see chapter 6.)

When you are involved in sports, naturally you perspire. Your body is cooled in this way and hurtful wastes are carried away. Sunscreens tend to retard perspiration and increase skin temperature, especially in climates marked by low humidity. Nevertheless, a Texas study has shown that it is safe to apply sunscreen liberally and often, especially after swimming or perspiring profusely. If it is very hot, exercise early in the morning or in the late afternoon.

Swimming and Its Associated Skin Problems

For many of us, summer means swimming. For the skin specialist, swimming means skin problems. Problems differ for those who swim in the ocean or a pool instead of fresh water. The first problem caused by water of any type is that it washes away natural skin oils as well as protective sunscreens (if they are not waterproof). Be sure to reapply your sunscreen after swimming. Sundown (Johnson & Johnson) is a waterproof sunscreen that resists washing off, but you should still touch up coverage after extended periods in the water.

Saltwater Exposure

Wash off salt after swimming in the ocean. Exposure to salt water affects the skin in a manner similar to vigorous perspiration. Salt dried on the skin actually draws moisture from the skin's surface, causing irritation and making skin more vulnerable. This can exacerbate eczema or other skin problems; exposure to sunlight only compounds any other skin damage.

Pool Problems

Swimmers often complain about the high levels of chlorine in pools, but without this disinfectant water easily becomes contaminated with disease-causing organisms. People are the main source of that contamination. Just one swimmer swimming continuously in a pool for one hour can deposit up to three pints of perspiration into the water. That perspiration serves as food for any microorganisms in the water and attracts bacteria in the pool just as perspiration attracts hungry bacteria on the surface of the body. Some basics for pool swimming are:

- Avoid cloudy pool water.
- Use the toilet before swimming.
- Shower before swimming.
- Stay away from pools altogether if you have boils or abcesses.

Although using a disinfectant foot bath before getting into any pool used to be considered mandatory, according to a study, it is worthless.

The chlorine used as a disinfectant and algicide in most pools is a powerful chemical that easily forms compounds with other materials, including protein. It bonds with hair and skin and is irritating. Reactions to chlorine are rarely allergic; they are generally just irritations. Chlorine is also more drying in conjunction with salt water, sun exposure, and perfumes.

Wash pool water from your skin and shampoo pool-wet hair as soon as you can. While still damp from the swim and your shower, smooth a small amount of a sunscreen-containing moisturizer all over your body as a barrier against further moisture loss.

Swimmer's Itch

Bathers who fancy the freshwater lakes of the Midwest—Wisconsin, Michigan, and Minnesota—often fall victim to periodic attacks of parasites that cause red bumps and itchy eruptions. Sea bathers suffer a saltwater version of the same problem. Both rashes appear on areas that have not been covered by the bathing suit. To prevent them, wash and dry thoroughly after swimming, and rub the body lightly with an astringent or alcohol. If you do get swimmer's itch, calamine lotion and an antihistamine will curb the symptoms.

Bikini Bottom

Wearing a wet bathing suit all day, especially if you are sitting on it, can cause an irritation of the hair follicles and the development of annoying pimples (folliculitis). The remedy seems obvious: After swimming and showering, put on dry clothes—or a dry bikini in place of the wet one if you want to remain on the beach. Using an absorbent powder such as Polysporin Powder (Burroughs Wellcome) will also help. If it is too late for prevention, you can try using antibiotic sprays—for example, Polysporin Spray—or antibotic creams topically.

Hot Tub Dermatitis

The increasing popularity of Jacuzzis, hot tubs, and whirlpools has given rise to a new form of infectious dermatitis, caused by bacteria that are able to survive high temperatures and chlorine levels.

Hot tub dermatitis is more likely to occur if chlorination of the tub or pool is inadequate and too many people are using the facility. (The New York State Health Code suggests that bather density be limited to one hot tub user per 25 square feet.) Too much time spent in the tub makes you more vulnerable to the bacteria there, and increased sweating and wet skin make it easier for the bacteria to penetrate. Skin abrasions also make bacterial invasion easier.

The itchy rash of hot tub dermatitis, which resembles insect bites, appears from eight hours to four days after exposure on the sides of the trunk and extremities (the areas that rub against the walls of the tub). Although the face and neck are usually spared, the infection can cause itchy eyes and ears as well as fatigue, sore throat, fever, nausea, vomiting, and abdominal cramps.

No treatment is required for this condition, which usually lasts about two weeks but sometimes longer than a month. Recurrences are possible.

To help prevent hot tub infections, shower and soap your body thoroughly with an antibacterial soap such as Safeguard after leaving the tub. Any vaginal discharge, itching, soreness of the eyes, or a runny nose that occurs a day or two after a session in the tub is cause for concern. If symptoms persist, consult your physician.

Stings and Bites

Water Creatures

Those who swim in the ocean or just walk along the shore may experience the painfully burning sting of jellyfish or stingrays. Jellyfish can sting several hours after they die—they wash up on the beach and lie in wait there for the unwary. The following creatures in particular have been recorded as biting or causing skin irritation to swimmers or fishermen who come in contact with them.

Sea urchins	Octopuses	Eels
Starfish	Squid	Catfish

If you are stung by a water creature, don't rub your skin or scratch it, as this only releases more toxins. Carefully treat the affected area as follows:

- Wash the area with sea water (not fresh water).
- Remove any tentacles.
- Soak the area in a weak solution of ammonia, alcohol, vinegar, or Burow's solution to neutralize the toxins. (Ice compresses retard absorption; warm or even hot compresses destroy jellyfish venom.)
- Apply unseasoned meat tenderizer: If you don't have any, apply salt, baking soda, flour, talc, or dry sand to absorb some of the toxins.

Many sea creatures produce a small capsule with a barb inside that sticks to the skin without being activated. The barb can be triggered some time later, often by fresh water—for example, in your shower. Sea urchins can leave their spines broken off in or underneath your skin, causing a severe burning and swelling or itching and redness that can be treated with applications of moist dressings, topical antibiotics, and antihistamines taken by mouth. If you can see the spine or barb, remove it carefully. A secondary reaction that may appear months later is the formation of a flesh-colored growth or bump.

A general rule for dealing with sea creatures is: Don't touch them. Their stings ordinarily produce little more than annoyance, but occasionally serious reactions to the toxins are reported. Corals, sea urchins, sponges, sea anemones, and certain other creatures are best left alone.

Keep rubber shoes on if you are walking on rocky or coral reefs. Besides protecting you from possible stings or bites, they will protect you from the danger of cuts from sharp rocks, coral, or shells.

Insect Stings and Bites

Mosquitos, blackflies, horseflies, bees, wasps, hornets, and—whether they fly or not—ants are the bane of campers and hikers. Their stings or bites, inflicted only by the females, can be serious or even lethal.

Honeybees leave their stingers and venom sacs in the skin. Remove the barbed stinger by scraping gently (use the dull side of a knife); impatiently plucking it out can release more venom.

The bites of insects are followed by a stinging pain; the damaged area can become swollen and itchy. The best relief is an immediate application of a paste made from equal parts of water and unseasoned meat tenderizer. Cold compresses may reduce swelling. You can also apply clear nail polish to the bite area (especially effective for chigger bites).

Recommended over-the-counter remedies include:

- Sarna Lotion (Stiefel)
- Prax Cream and Lotion (Ferndale)
- Eurax Cream and Lotion (Westwood)—by prescription

If the symptoms are severe, see your dermatologist. Antihistamines or cortisone-based drugs may be necessary. If you suffer a severe allergic reaction, use an asthma-relief inhaler as a temporary measure until you can get medical help. Most important, try not to scratch. Irritating the skin further can leave you open to secondary infections.

You can defend yourself against flying insects by making yourself less obvious as a target: Wear light, neutral-colored clothing and avoid glittery jewelry, perfumes, and hair sprays. Sweet scents attract insects—some people seem naturally to smell sweeter to insects than others. Using an absorbent powder to stay dry also helps. Vitamin B_1, garlic, and onions have some insect-repelling abilities. Repellents containing DEET are helpful— liquid products have higher concentrations of the active ingredient. Using a couple of different types of repellents at once is usually more effective than using just one.

Poison Ivy

A perfect example of allergic contact dermatitis is the reaction of many persons (if they are sensitive) to poison ivy, poison oak, or poison sumac. The areas most commonly affected are the extremities, neck, and face, although the typical redness, blisters, and swelling occur wherever the plant's oily sap from the leaves or stem contacts the skin. If the area around the eyes is involved, there can be severe swelling.

You can be affected by oil that has been picked up from contacts with the plants and transported on animal coats, your own clothing, or sporting equipment. Even smoke from a garden fire can bring with it the burning and itching of poison ivy. The ooze from the blisters doesn't spread the rash, but the oil from the plant itself does if hands or clothing are contaminated. Though it is more common in the summer, you can get poison ivy any time of the year if you are in an area where it grows. If you have had poison ivy before, it will take only a couple of days after exposure for the rash to appear. If you are reacting for the first time, it can take two weeks or even longer.

If you are allergic to poison ivy, learn to recognize the plant's appearance and stay away from it. Wear clothing that covers arms and legs if you are in a high-risk area. If you think you have been exposed to the plant, take a shower within fifteen minutes, and then take frequent very warm showers for that first day. If you can't get to a shower, at least try to wash your hands and exposed areas with soap immediately. Contaminated clothing, including shoes, should be washed with detergent or dry-cleaned.

Folk remedies include applications of grated potato, washing with laundry soap, and touching the area with roll-on deodorant. None of these has been shown to be effective.

Here are some better treatment options:

- Try cool compresses of Burow's solution (Domeboro). Use them for ten minutes at four-hour intervals.
- Witch hazel, calamine lotion, or over-the-counter hydrocortisone cream or lotion such as Cortaid (Upjohn) applied two or three times a day are helpful in mild cases.
- Oral antihistamines such as Chlor-Trimeton (Schering) or Benadryl (Parke-Davis) will help stop itching and calm skin.
- A soothing warm bath with Aveeno Oilated (Cooper) can also help.

If the rash is severe, a dermatologist can administer cortisone injections or prescribe a short course of oral steroids supplemented by antihistamine tablets to relieve the itching.

Heat Rash

Heat rash, also called prickly heat or miliaria, is caused by an obstruction of the sweat ducts that afflicts some women in hot weather. It is usually seen as multiple tiny red bumps on the skin.

An excellent remedy for prickly heat is a cool colloidal oatmeal bath:

1. Run a tub of cool to lukewarm water.
2. Put a tablespoon of raw oatmeal in the middle of a thin cotton

handkerchief. Knot the handkerchief to prevent the oatmeal from leaking out.

3. Place the oatmeal packet in your tub. Get in and relax for about ten minutes.
4. After drying sprinkle yourself with body powder. I like Youth-Dew Dusting Powder from Estée Lauder. If you are allergic to fragrances, use a nonscented product such as Johnson's Baby Powder or talcum powder. (For more about heat rash, see chapter 24.)

Cold-Weather Sports and Skin

Outdoor sports, particularly jogging, can bring on specific skin problems.

Windburn and chapping are a serious problem in cold-weather sports. The skin becomes dehydrated, rough, and flaky. Thick, oily, and occlusive protection is needed. Cyclists and skiers subjected to cold winds find it important to cover the face, hands, and even hair to prevent the loss of moisture. Look for products that are formulated to protect especially sensitive areas such as the eyelids, lips, and ears from harsh climatic conditions. Don't forget to use sunscreen.

Chapped hands bother almost everyone: Apply moisturizer at least fifteen minutes before going out. Using a double layer of gloves—cotton or silk under leather or wool—will protect the skin of your hands better than wearing a single pair and will also keep your fingers warmer.

Exercise increases circulation to the hands and feet. Keep active—wiggle your fingers and toes, jump up and down, and rotate your arms at the shoulders.

Loose, warm, layered clothing helps to prevent damage to skin. Down, fur, foam, and wool are best for preserving body heat.

Staying dry is almost as important as staying warm; evaporation will cool the body very quickly. Change damp clothing immediately.

Frostbite and Frost Nip

Like a burn, frostbite is an injury that may result in the loss of tissue. Its severity is determined in part by the temperature and also by the humidity and wind velocity at the time of exposure. When the skin of the nose, toes, fingers, or ears turns yellow or whitish, don't ignore the problem—what you do can make a big difference in recovery. A moderate frost nip can quickly become a severe frostbite. If you are not sure of how to treat frostbite yourself, try to find someone who does know how to treat it. Prompt and informed treatment can help. The wrong treatment can be harmful.

- Avoid alcoholic drinks. They numb sensation in the affected areas and sensitivity of feeling in the affected areas is a guide to treatment.
- Warm frostbitten areas rapidly but *gently*. Beware of scalding or

burning numb tissue. Warm hands and feet in a blanket or in lukewarm (*not* hot) water.

• Cover a frostbitten nose with your fingers; tuck frostbitten fingers under your arms.
• Do not massage or rub the affected areas; this can cause damage.
• Once these preliminary procedures have been followed, get to a physician as soon as possible.

If you are a jogger who listens to music through headphones while jogging, be aware that metal earplugs can transmit cold. Use rubber earplugs or a hat or headband between skin and metal earplugs.

Sports-Related Allergic Reactions

Just as some people develop allergies to work conditions, they actually can develop allergies to exercise (in the form of hives)! Hives, or urticaria, can be caused by a number of factors, including friction due to tight clothing or any other kind of pressure, sun, heat, cold air or water, and—occasionally—chlorine.

If hives are due to heat or related causes, Benadryl capsules (Parke-Davis) will help. For hives that are a reaction to cold, your dermatologist can prescribe a different antihistamine. Use this test to determine whether you have cold urticaria: Place an ice cube on your forearm for fifteen minutes. If you are afflicted, the area will become red, swollen, start to itch, and develop welts.

Fungal Infections

Athlete's Foot

Athlete's foot, or tinea pedis, has long been a common complaint among sports enthusiasts. More men than women are affected, and more young than old (it occurs most frequently between the ages of fifteen and forty). In recent years, as more women have dedicated themselves to exercise and thus come to frequent locker rooms and wear sneakers or running shoes, the incidence of athlete's foot among women has increased. At least 90 percent of all adults have mild fungal infections between their toes.

Some believe that everyone is a potential candidate for athlete's foot because the fungi causing it are always around, but that an active infection will appear only when the natural resistance of the skin is lowered. Friction, sweaty toes that don't get enough ventilation, and dirty, perspiration-laden socks all lower resistance.

Severe athlete's foot outbreaks are caused by several different types of fungal organisms, including yeast and molds. These types of fungi thrive in warm, moist, alkaline areas like the toe webs. (A fungus cannot survive on an acid surface.) The rash may be itchy, red, and scaling; the toe webs may appear white and soggy, and white scales are common between the fourth and fifth toes.

Another common form of athlete's foot consists of a dry scaling on the entire sole in a moccasin pattern. Treat it as you would regular athlete's foot.

Fighting Athlete's Foot

Athlete's foot is usually fairly easy to treat, but at times it can be stubborn. The wrong over-the-counter medications may actually aggravate your condition. If you have a persistent foot rash, consult your dermatologist, who in severe cases is likely to prescribe antifungal medication to be taken orally. It takes time, about four weeks, to make headway against a savage case of athlete's foot, so don't be discouraged. Some over-the-counter products are:

- Desenex (Pharmacraft)
- Footwork (Lederle)
- Zeasorb-AF (Stiefel)
- Micatin (Ortho)
- Tinactin (Schering)
- Aftate (Plough)

If you use an antifungal powder, you can avoid the mess of loose powder by putting it in a plastic or paper bag, then putting your foot in the bag and shaking it all about.

Prevention, of course, is the best treatment. Follow these preventive measures to keep fungus away:

- Wash your feet daily, rinse well, and dry them carefully and completely with a towel, and then allow them to air-dry for five to ten minutes before putting on your socks and shoes. To speed complete drying, hold a hair dryer about six inches from your foot, wiggle your toes, and dry between them.
- Before you put on socks or hose, sprinkle some antiperspirant foot powder between your toes. Use the powder sparingly to avoid caking.
- Wear only clean cotton socks, not socks made with synthetic yarns. Make sure that they have been rinsed thoroughly during laundering— any residue of detergent will aggravate your skin problem. Natural materials such as cotton and leather create the best environment for the feet, while rubber and wool may induce sweating and hold moisture.
- Avoid tight, snug, or unventilated footwear. Don't wear boots all day; wear sandals in the summer when possible. Plastic shoes and boots are fun and great as rainwear but serve as hotels for fungal infections.
- Wiggle your toes to let air circulate between your toes.
- Avoid walking barefoot through gyms, spas, health clubs, and locker rooms—even around swimming pools. Fungal infections can be picked up almost anyplace that is damp if you are prone to them.

Not every skin reaction on the foot is athlete's foot, of course; rashes and irritations can also represent contact dermatitis—that is, allergic reactions to the shoes that the athlete wears. Plastic or rubber shoes that keep the feet moist and don't allow ventilation, the curing agent in leather shoes, or the dye used to finish the leather all can be at fault.

Athlete's Toenails

Toenails are also often infected by the fungi that cause athlete's foot. The nail thickens and becomes yellowish with crumbly material accumulating under the nail. Toenail infections are notoriously resistant to topical treatment. An oral antifungal medication must be used, but the infection may recur even after a year of treatment. Once the infection is cured, topical treatments may be used to prevent reinfection.

Jock Itch—For Jocks of Either Sex

Another fungal infection that torments the athlete leads to a light brown or reddish eruption with a sharp scaling border that follows the folds of the skin where it is warm and moist, notably in the groin. The diagnosis and treatment of this fungal infection, tinea cruris, is similar to that for athlete's foot.

Jock itch is more common in men, but women can get it, particularly if they are overweight. The rash is associated with a burning itch and can spread to thighs if left untreated.

Once infected with jock itch, you may expect a cure to be effective in about two weeks. Effective over-the-counter products include:

- Micatin (Ortho)
- Tinactin (Schering)
- Cruex (Pharmacraft)
- Vioform (Ciba)

Follow these preventive measures to keep the groin free of fungi:

- Keep the area dry.
- Powder the area with talc or cornstarch (avoid scented powders since you might be allergic to their perfume).
- Favor loose, absorbent cotton clothing.

Intertrigo

Intertrigo, although not caused by a fungus, is often confused with jock itch and can lead to a fungal infection. It is a superficial dermatitis that occurs in folds of the skin. Joggers sometimes experience it in the form of a red, macerated rash on the delicate skin of the inner thigh or under the breast. The condition can also develop from the irritation of a bicycle seat or a saddle used in horseback riding. The rash itself is not serious, but the irritated skin invites a more serious fungal or bacterial infection. The best way to soothe the irritation is to reduce friction and keep the area dry.

In general, to avoid skin irritations of various kinds, keep the skin cool and firm. The fewer skin folds you have, the less chance you have that any area will remain continuously moist from perspiration or washing or be irritated by friction. This constitutes just one more argument for staying slim and trim.

Tinea Versicolor

A very common fungal infection, tinea versicolor is usually associated with warmer weather and generally affects young people. The condition is caused by an overgrowth of the yeast that normally lives on the skin, and there appears to be a genetic predisposition to the infection. Tinea versicolor is a multicolored rash that can range from yellow to reddish to brown. It appears on the chest, back, neck, and, if not treated, the abdomen, arms, thighs, and legs. (Blacks may get the rash on the face as well.)

Most people notice the condition only after having been in the sun for a while because the fungus acts as a sunscreen, preventing affected areas from getting darker—so the rash appears as light spots. The condition is unattractive but not dangerous and usually has no related symptoms. However, when victims perspire the spots can become angry, red, and itchy, and if the condition is not treated, it will spread (recurrences are common). If you have been diagnosed as having tinea versicolor, there are some home remedies:

- Try using benzoyl peroxide or sulfur/salicylic acid soap with a Buf-Puf or loofah. In mild cases this will peel enough of the skin to get rid of the fungus.
- Shampoos containing zinc pyrithione (Zincon/Lederle) or selenium sulfide (Selsun Blue/Ross) can be applied to the body with a paintbrush. Do this every day for thirty days, letting the shampoo stay on for thirty minutes, or twice a week for two weeks with the shampoo left on overnight. In severe cases, a physician may prescribe Selsun lotion (Abbott).
- Tinver (Barnes-Hind) and Micatin (Ortho Pharmaceutical) are two over-the-counter antifungal agents that can be used twice a day for two weeks. Antifungal creams available by prescription include Loprox (Hoechst-Roussel), Spectasole (Ortho Pharmaceutical), and Mycelex (Miles Pharmaceutical). In stubborn cases Ketoconazole tablets (Janssen) may be prescribed.

Friction Problems

Almost any sport can cause friction—devotees of exercise classes suffer mat burns, and bowlers suffer finger calluses. Here are some of the problems that may result from friction.

Calluses

If mild friction—not enough to form a blister—constantly irritates an area of the skin, the skin gradually thickens and a callus is formed. If the friction continues over a long period of time, as happens when one makes continuous use of a paddle, bow, or tennis racket, the callus can get very thick. Many foot calluses are more than half an inch thick, and hand calluses from the use of weight-training machines sometimes are also quite impressive. Gymnastics, rowing, and golf are only a few of the sports that encourage calluses. Plantar calluses—thickenings of the skin of the soles—are frequently brought on by high heels. Men and women who wear only flat shoes seldom have plantar calluses, although these calluses can also be caused by the sliding and shifting of weight inside a sports shoe or sneaker.

Many sportspersons find that the area of the callus is less sensitive. The lack of sensitivity can throw off your tennis serve or ruin your golf swing, but it can also allow you to exercise for longer periods of time. Depending on your perspective, the callus can be regarded as either an unwanted growth or a wanted cushion.

You can rid yourself of calluses this way:

1. Soak the area in warm water.
2. Gently rub the area with a pumice stone or abrasive to wear down the dead skin. (Repeat several times a week, preferably daily.)
3. Apply moisturizer containing urea or lactic acid or both.

The best time to rub calluses away is after bathing, because hydrated skin responds best to the pumice treatment. For more stubborn calluses try a premedicated skin pad of 40 percent salicylic acid plaster.

Feet and hands are not the only areas of the body subject to enough wear to develop calluses. Horseback and bicycle riders sometimes develop calluses on the insides of the knees or on their buttocks. These can be treated the same way.

Corns

When a toe rubs against a shoe or is out of line with the others, it may become irritated. The repeated friction increases the blood supply, which in turn accelerates cell production of a cornified substance—and a corn develops to protect the toe. Corns are usually smaller than calluses.

You can treat a corn at home. First find out what is causing the problem—a badly fitted shoe or some other friction—and then try applying moleskin to prevent or reduce friction between the shoe and the toe. You can use an over-the-counter corn remover, but use it very cautiously. Don't deviate from the directions or you can damage unaffected areas of the skin.

Plantar Warts

Plantar calluses seem predisposed to invasion by the wart virus, resulting in plantar warts. Perspiration plays a role in their development, so athletes are more prone to them. Because it grows up into the foot, a plantar wart can be quite painful. If you have a wart, wear comfortable shoes with pads to reduce the pressure on it.

To treat a plantar wart, soak your foot in hot water, then cover the wart with a salicylic acid pad such as Mediplast (Beiersdorf), which is a 40 percent salicylic acid plaster. Carefully smooth the wart's surface with an emery board. Alternate salicylic acid pads with Verucid gel (Ulmer). Don't be impatient. Even with prescription-strength preparations a plantar wart may require more than three weeks of treatment. Surgery is sometimes necessary for stubborn warts.

Thinning Hair

Gymnasts, yoga enthusiasts, and break dancers experience problems with thinning hair because of constant rubbing on the top of their scalp during headstands. Weight trainers sometimes notice a thinning of hair caused by friction on the back of the head against a padded support. Wearing earphones, especially during jogging when the headband rubs against the scalp and breaks hair, can cause hair thinning along the band. Happily, hair loss of this sort can be reversed by abandoning the activity.

Runner's Nipples

Women joggers should wear a bra or cover their nipples with Band-Aids and apply lubricants to avoid the irritation known as runner's nipples. This condition can range from peeling to sores.

No matter what your exercise or sport, you will move better, feel more comfortable, and suffer fewer skin and other problems if what you wear closest to your skin is right. A sports bra is a skin-care must for most women. Although women with small breasts can probably wear any soft seamless bra for workouts, a specially designed sports bra is advisable for anyone with more than an A-cup size. A sports bra should minimize breast movement. Besides promoting runner's nipples, bouncing can break down fragile breast support tissue and cause the breasts to sag.

Black Heel, Black Palm, and Blue Toe

Tennis, racquet ball, squash, and handball are wonderful for building stamina and mobility, but they all can lead to *talon noir,* or black heel, an irregular bluish black discoloration at the heel caused by stop-and-go and back-and-forth action. Any sport that gives the heel a pounding can cause capillaries to break or leak, and then the blood appears under the skin as purplish black.

Black palm, often called biker's palm, is similar. It appears on the hands and is attributed to a sudden lateral shearing force that causes hemorrhaging under the skin's surface. Black heel and black palm will both gradually disappear without treatment.

Constant pressure, slamming, and jarring damages toes, too. Fast stops crush the toe against the front of your sports shoe, causing bending of the nail and bleeding underneath it—blue, or tennis, toe. The second toe of tennis players, the large toe of those who play other racquet sports, the third toe of soccer players, and the fourth and fifth toes of joggers are most frequently affected.

The best treatment is prevention: Wear carefully fitted shoes and thick socks that act as shock absorbers. If a blue nail does develop, however, here is what to do:

1. Relieve pressure on the nail by cutting away the toe area of your shoe.
2. Cut the nail as short as possible.
3. Soak in warm water twice a day.
4. Insert a protective guard inside your shoe.

If you ignore the problem, your nail can eventually fall off. Play it safe: Make sure your skin and nails are protected. A physician may have to evacuate blood accumulated under the nail.

If you suffer numbness and weakness in your palms after regularly riding a bicycle, the problem may be with the handlebar pressure on a nerve in the palm. Cover your handlebar with extra padding on the palm area, and change hand position often when you are on a long ride.

Exercise Acne

Friction can cause acne on the forehead and shoulders, where oil glands are concentrated. Exercise acne is caused by friction of tight clothing, especially when it gets wet or there is excessive perspiration. Leather and cloth headbands can rub in perspiration. Even friction with sporting equipment can be a contributing factor. The combination of pressure, friction, heat, and perspiration stimulates the release of oil and leads to acne by occluding the follicular openings. Perspiration is comedogenic—pores are more easily blocked when skin is covered with sweat.

To prevent exercise acne:

• Wear loose-fitting cotton clothing.
• Change clothing as soon as it gets wet.
• Keep hair away from your face while exercising.
• Use an alcohol-based astringent on the face immediately after exercising; use a mechanical cleanser such as Buf-Puf on susceptible areas; use an abrasive soap on the body.
• Be sure your cleanly laundered sports clothes and headbands are thoroughly rinsed to remove detergent residue.

Hair Care for Sports

Too much exposure to the sun and wind when golfing, swimming, skiing, or playing tennis can create serious health problems for your hair. Jacob Neal, hairdresser to the Ladies Professional Golf Association, says that since a golfer's head remains in the same position for a long time, the hair on the crown of her head becomes particularly sun-damaged. The hair sometimes loses its elasticity and won't curl at all. The same problem can affect anyone who is motionless in the sun for long periods of time. Conditioners should be applied to the crown of the head as well as the hair ends.

Hair can also be sun-damaged when skiing. Aspen and other high-mountain ski centers are located at altitudes of almost two miles—the sun cuts through less atmosphere on its way to the Earth and thus can more forcefully bleach and dry the hair. Dry and flaky scalp conditions as well as frozen and brittle split ends are all improved by the application of conditioners.

Women who play indoor sports such as racquet ball or use health clubs have hair problems, too. Dry indoor air and the jouncing your hair takes as you bounce around the gym can loosen curls or cause your hair to go frizzy. The dry/wet cycle also plays havoc with any set; keeping hair restrained can help preserve it a little longer.

Swimmer's Hair

Salt water speeds up the oxidation process that affects colored hair. If you color your hair, you will find that swimming bareheaded in the ocean means you have to color more often—always a trauma for hair. Exposure to salt water also strips natural oils from hair, leaves deposits on hair and scalp, and damages permanents. The chlorinated water in swimming pools can damage your hair as well.

No one seems to wear bathing caps anymore, but everyone should. Caps help to:

- Preserve body heat, especially if you swim for long periods of time in the ocean, or in a cold mountain lake
- Protect against dry, brittle hair and scalp irritations caused by pool disinfectants
- Defend against green-tinged hair due to copper used in pools to retard the growth of algae

To prevent swimmer's hair, rinse hair in fresh water immediately after swimming (adding a teaspoon of baking soda to the water helps remove residue of chlorine).

If wearing a cap is too confining or unstylish for you, you can still usually keep your hair in top form by:

- Shampooing immediately after swimming with a mild, oily castile shampoo or a special swimmer's shampoo that breaks the bond chlorine forms with the proteins in your skin and hair
- Using a hot oil treatment to help remove tints and keep hair soft
- Patting, squeezing, and wrapping your hair until it's drip-free
- Allowing your hair to air-dry without combing or brushing. (The less you do to wet hair, the better.)

Copper is deposited more easily on treated or colored hair, especially blond, silvery, or light hair. If you find your hair discolored, you can bring it back to a natural shade by rinsing it in a weak (3 percent) solution of hydrogen peroxide, leaving the rinse on the hair for two to three hours. Consistent use of Revlon's Ultra Swim shampoo over a period of a few weeks can also erase the greenish tinge.

Some other aids for damaged color-treated hair:

- Rub heated vegetable oil into your hair and let it stay on for fifteen minutes.

- Deep-condition your hair every other week; this can diminish the greenish tinge.
- For very severe cases, products containing EDTA (ethylenediamine tetra-acetate)—such as Nexus Aloe Clarifier (Jheri Redding)—left on for thirty minutes will bring your hair back to its color.

A Conditioning Program for Athletic Hair

Hot olive oil works very well as a conditioner for athletic hair. It can be applied to the hair every fifth or sixth shampoo (for some women athletes that means every few days) in the following way:

1. Pour about 1/4 cup of olive oil into a juice glass or other narrow glass container. Set this in a larger glass of very hot water for about fifteen minutes.
2. While you wait for the oil to warm, brush your hair, bending low from the waist and gently massaging your scalp. Start at the back of the neck and brush down toward the hairline at your forehead.
3. Apply the warm oil to the scalp and work it through the hair to the ends.
4. Wrap the hair in Saran Wrap or in a plastic bag or cap. Allow the warm oil to stay on the hair for about ten minutes (longer will not hurt).
5. Wash the hair carefully, shampooing several times. Rinse in cool water.

The stress of competition triggers a change in the balance of hormones within some women and increases the oil secretions on the skin and in the scalp. If you find exercise makes your hair oilier, use the hot oil only on the hair ends. (Usually hair ends are dry no matter how oily the scalp is.)

Dandruff affects businesswomen tense from working under high pressure, and women athletes performing under the pressure of severe competition have the same problem. Follow the guidelines in chapter 13 if you experience a problem with dandruff.

Exercise and Makeup

If you are concerned enough about your appearance to be staying in shape, chances are you want to look good while exercising. Some tips on wearing makeup while active:

- Keep makeup to a minimum.
- When exercising outdoors, always use a water-resistant sunscreen.
- Do not overmoisturize. *Do* opt for an oil-free moisturizer.
- Wearing foundation is not a good idea, but if you must, make sure that it is water-based and oil-free (top with loose powder to set).
- Use waterproof mascara and powder eye shadows and blushers.
- Use lipsticks with sunscreen added.

Sports and Skin Care at a Glance

Winter Sports

Skiing	Ice skating
Tobogganing	Cross-country skiing

What to Wear

To retain body heat most effectively, dress warmly in layers of loose clothing. Natural fibers that do not adjust rapidly to the temperature of the environment are best. Protect your face with a scarf or ski mask. Use lip balms and heavy occlusive moisturizers that contain sunscreen.

What to Watch For

Avoid direct contact of exposed skin with metal, which transmits cold. If tingling, burning, and pain are followed by numbness, it could mean frost nip or frostbite. Gently immerse the affected part in a water bath at the temperature of 104°F to 110°F. Never rub the affected part with anything, including snow. If blisters develop, apply wet compresses. See your physician: Frostbite can be serious.

Gymnasium Sports

Martial arts	Boxing	Ballet
Wrestling	Fencing	Jazz dancing
Aerobic dancing		

What to Wear

Light natural-fiber clothing that will allow movement and absorb perspiration. Keep muscles warm with layers of knitted garments. Keep sports clothing clean.

What to Watch For

Beware mat burns and blisters. Herpes simplex (cold sores) and other viral and bacterial infections can be passed via body contact.

Equipment Sports

Bodybuilding	Weight training

What to Wear

Cloth and leather headbands often worn during sweat-inducing exercises can combine with friction to trigger acne. Keep such bands clean, or better yet, do without them. Wear soft, absorbent fabrics—cotton is best. Wear only pristine shirts.

What to Watch For

Irritation from sweat and rubbing against cycle seats, padded bars, and other equipment can encourage jock itch and other sweat-related skin irritations. Heavy straps and padded equipment can also be the home of bacteria and fungi. Wash very carefully after exercising, and make sure your health club lives up to its health code. Wear rubber sandals in locker rooms.

Stop-and-Go Sports

Racquet ball	Tennis	Squash	Handball
Paddle ball	Volleyball	Basketball	Field hockey

What to Wear

Properly fitted shoes are vital to good performance and safety. Purchase them at a sporting goods store that stocks a variety of athletic shoes, and make sure the salesperson knows what sport you plan to use them for.

What to Watch For

The wrong or poorly fitted shoes can cause blisters, calluses, plantar warts, and tennis toes. They also can be responsible for twisted ankles and falls.

Outdoor Activities

Hiking	Walking	Camping
Rowing	Climbing	Golf
Cycling	Horseback riding	Roller skating

What to Wear

Wear light- or medium-toned pastel clothing and no perfume (to avoid attracting insects). Carefully fitting the shoulder straps of a backpack to distribute weight and pressure evenly can prevent blisters on your shoulders or body. Changing socks frequently is a must for walkers and hikers.

What to Watch For

Carry extra protective clothing and sunscreen. Stop and rest often—accidents happen when you are tired.

Water Sports

Swimming	Water-skiing
Diving	Scuba diving

What to Wear

Sunscreen, sunscreened lip balm, and sunblock. Certain fabric dyes, especially blues, are photosensitizing and can, if used in swimsuits, encourage sunburn under the suit. Wet T-shirts offer almost no protection.

What to Watch For

You can get burned on a cloudy day, under water (less than 10 feet), and through glass. Be prepared.

13

HOW TO MAINTAIN
YOUR SHINY MANE

To know yourself you must know your hair; it mirrors your inner health and outer self. Shiny, clean hair is a high status accessory as well as an important frame for the face. Dull, drab hair, overprocessed hair, or limp, lifeless, or brassy tresses announce something is wrong—no matter what garments you're wearing or how perfect your complexion or makeup may be.

My hair is my best feature, and I enjoy taking care of it. When my hair is freshly clean, colored, and set, I feel glorious; when it is lank and dark-rooted, nothing can raise my spirits. One of my patients with oily hair described her sufferings vividly: "It makes me feel like putting my head in a bag. I dread seeing anyone I know."

Lively Hair Is Dead

The hair we see is nonliving. It is actually similar to nails in structure, and like nails it is composed of 98 percent protein in a substance called keratin. The keratin of the horny layer or outermost surface of the skin is called soft keratin, and it sloughs away easily and naturally. Hair and nails are made up of hard keratin, which has a higher sulfur content.

Hair is produced in the follicles within the skin; each follicle produces a single strand of hair. Each hair has three separate layers:

1. The outer coating of the hair is called the cuticle. It is very much like the horny layer of the skin. It is colorless and protective and contributes to the strength of the hair.
2. The middle layer is the cortex. It contains the pigment that colors the hair. The cortex is mainly responsible for hair's strength, diameter, and configuration.
3. The innermost layer of the hair is called the medulla. Its function is somewhat mysterious, although it is believed to bring oxygen to the hair and influence its color.

How Hair Grows

The hair-forming cells in the follicles work for about three years, producing strands of hair each about a yard long (the length it would be if you were not to cut it). The follicles then go into a three-month rest period. At the end of this period, the hair falls out. Each hair has its own life-span, and hair follicles function asynchronically.

On any day 100 of the approximately 100,000 hairs in your scalp fall away. Daily loss of these 100 or so hairs is a normal process. A new hair soon grows to replace each fallen hair—and the cycle begins again.

The three stages of this growth-rest-shed cycle are:

1. *Anagen* (growth). This stage lasts from three to ten years (the longer it lasts, the longer hair grows). During this phase activity in the hair follicle is great, contributing to the length and diameter of the hair shaft. Eighty to 90 percent of the hair on your scalp is in the growing stage. The average rate of growth is two inches per three months. Anticancer drugs (chemotherapy), radiation, and some endocrine diseases can end the anagen stage of growth.
2. *Catagen* (transition to rest). This stage lasts about three weeks. It signals a stopping of any activity in the follicle, including pigment production.
3. *Telogen* (resting/falling). During the resting phase the follicle shrinks, the hair loosens in the follicle, then it falls from the follicle. This resting/falling stage lasts three to five months. Some hair loss is temporary and some is permanent.

High fever, stress, and faulty diet are some of the reasons for temporary hair loss. When a new hair fails to grow in the empty follicle, there is a permanent hair loss. Generally 10 to 20 percent of hair on the scalp is in the resting/falling stage at any one time.

Age, changes in hormones, and faulty diet can shorten the growth cycle and increase the rest cycle, slowing hair growth. Growth noticeably declines between the ages of about fifty and sixty, which accounts for postmenopausal thinning hair.

Women's hair usually grows faster than men's hair and grows most luxuriantly between the ages of fifteen and thirty. Hair grows fastest during summer. More hair falls out in the fall. The last trimester of pregnancy is also a period of rapid hair growth.

Why Hair Is Thin or Thick

Thick hair is full, luxurious, manageable, and strong (resistant to bending and breaking). When the length of the rest cycle increases and a greater than normal number of hairs stop growing, the hair gradually thins. At age twenty the average scalp has about 100,000 hairs, with about 700 in each square centimeter of scalp; at age fifty only about 500 are in the same area. If there are fewer than 400 hairs, the area is noticeably thin.

How do you know how many hairs you lose? Comb or brush your hair over a sheet of paper and place the hair in an envelope and date it (add any hair from your pillow or sink). Repeat the exercise several times over the course of several weeks. Then compare the contents of the envelopes to see if there is more or less hair day by day. Only a drastic difference should give you reason to worry. If you don't shampoo daily you will find that there is more hair lost on the days you wash it.

The thickness of your hair depends on:

- The number of follicles in your scalp
- The number of hairs that are growing from those follicles
- The diameter of the strands of hairs
- Genetic predisposition

Curly red hair needs only about 85,000 hairs to appear thick and luxuriant because red hair is thicker than either brown or blond hair, and curly hair is usually thicker and has more body than straight hair. Brunettes average about 100,000 hairs per scalp for a full look, while a blonde will need about 140,000 hairs because blond hair is usually fine and thin—in other words, has a smaller diameter. With age, hair of every color becomes smaller in diameter.

If you want thicker hair, you can color it. Coloring swells the cortex and raises the cuticle, making the hair diameter greater and the hair strands thicker. Or you can use thickening shampoos or conditioners that coat the strands of hair. (Don't use a thickening shampoo *and* conditioner; too much can leave hair limp.) The bases of these thickeners are waxes that add to the diameter of each hair strand. Two of these products are Thicket (Madric) and Thick'n Hair (Fantasia).

Beer, avocado, and egg yolk adhere to hair and can be used to add body. Hair sprays, setting lotions, mousses, and gels also increase hair's body. A shorter, blunt-cut hairstyle makes hair look thicker. (For more on why hair thins and how to treat it, see chapter 14.)

Texture

Hair texture often determines the perception of a woman's age. Texture refers to the degree of straightness or curl, the thickness of the individual hairs, and the look and feel of the hair. Hair often loses smoothness, bounce, and luster long before it goes gray. It changes many times during life:

- From ages one to five, baby curls may become straight.
- In puberty and adolescence, hair thickens and color changes.
- In the twenties and thirties, hair may become progressively curly or may go from curly to kinky.
- Gray hairs may begin appearing already in the twenties, although usually not in quantity until the forties or fifties. Gray hair differs substantially from other hair and is often wiry with a larger strand diameter than other hair.

Although hair texture follows hormonal changes in the body, there is no conclusive evidence that hormones are responsible for sudden hair texture changes in healthy women. The increase in oiliness during adolescence, when the weather is warmer, and during periods of stress affects only the surface feeling of the hair. However, the vitamin A derivative Accutane, used in treating acne, has been reported to make straight hair curly in some cases.

Straight or Curly?

The shape of the individual hair strands determines the straightness, waviness, or curliness of your hair:

- Straight hair is almost round.
- Wavy hair is oval.
- Curly hair is almost flat.

Flat, curly hair shafts have a tendency to grow at uneven rates and to grow unevenly in the follicle, first growing toward one side and then the other. Such hair seems to have a mind of its own. If wavy or curly hair is allowed to grow long, the weight of the strands will stretch the wave and the hair will appear straighter, but a natural tendency to curliness and curly traits remain.

Coarse Hair?

Very thick curly hair often feels coarse to the touch, stands away from the head, has little shine, and defies styling. Black hair sometimes has the properties typical of coarse hair. Don't confuse coarse hair with dry hair.

Coarse hair can be softened and the molecular bonds that keep it springy relaxed to make it more manageable and shiny. Using a hot comb can be very damaging to the hair shafts.

The most effective way to straighten hair is chemically. Thioglycollate, an alkaline solution that is also used in cold waving, is used to unwave. It softens the hair shaft. The drawback is that suddenly your hair will seem oily. The chemical process has not made the hair oily; it is only that natural oils now coat the hair more evenly and effectively. Hair treated in this way is also weaker, so avoid hot blow dryers. (For more about straightening hair see chapter 15.)

If you do not want to use a straightener, always potentially damaging to the hair, here is a program:

- Shampoo with a high-alkaline soapy product.
- Use a high-alkaline conditioner.
- Avoid vinegar or lemon rinses—they make the curl tighter by tightening the cuticle.
- Use a cream rinse and leave it on your hair as long as the directions indicate; you can heighten its effect by wrapping your hair in a plastic shower cap while the rinse is doing its work. Then rinse completely with clear, lukewarm water—this coats each strand, making it lank and slickly oily.
- Set your hair wet, and be sure it is completely dry before styling.

Shiny and Bouncy?

The hair's cuticle, its outer protective coating, is the most important layer when it comes to maintaining good condition. The cells of the cuticle are arranged in up to ten layers in shingle fashion. These cells are transparent, allowing the cortex to be seen and light to reflect off the hair shaft. The reflection of light off the cuticle is what makes the hair shine.

When hair is healthy, cuticle cells are flat, overlapping smoothly, reflecting light and making hair shiny. When the cells have been irritated or damaged, their edges curl up and stand away from the hair shaft. The smooth reflective surface is broken and the hair looks dull. With wear and tear the number of cuticle cells toward the ends of hairs also decreases and, if reduced completely, exposes the cortex.

Hair Oils and Shine

Oil glands in the scalp also play a part in keeping your hair shiny. As each hair grows it is coated with sebum, which prevents evaporation of moisture from the hair shaft. The oil also forms a reflective coating on the cuticle, which makes the strand shiny and fills any cracks so that each strand is smooth. While some women apply oils and pomades or dressings to make their hair look shiny, the result is usually an unnatural shine due to an excess of oil.

Hormones control the oil glands in the scalp in the same way they affect the oil glands on your face. When the androgen-estrogen balance is tipped toward the androgens, too much oil is secreted. Brushing distributes oil along the shaft and makes it look shiny, but brushing can also stimulate the oil glands and make hair more oily. Do your most vigorous brushing in the morning. Avoid overbrushing.

Softness of the skin and flexibility of the nails are due to their ability to absorb and hold water. The same is true for hair. Healthy hair contains enough water (10 to 20 percent) to keep its moistness. Moist hair is elastic; if you pull gently on it, it stretches but does not break. Dry hair (with less than 10 to 20 percent water) becomes brittle; it breaks or damages easily and it is dull.

Cuticle Damage and Dull Hair

Dull hair is often the result of cuticle damage, which can be caused by a variety of things:

- Excessive combing or brushing, especially when hair is wet
- Overwashing without conditioning, which lifts the cuticle
- Alkaline shampoos, which make the hair shaft swell and force away the cuticle
- Chemical processes such as bleaching, coloring, perming, or straightening, as well as using hot rollers or curling irons and brushes. These processes make the damaged cuticle more susceptible to other trauma.
- Rough towel drying, especially if the cuticle is already damaged
- External factors such as sunlight, heat, wind, and rain
- Prolonged pressure from hair elastics, barrettes, rollers, and wigs, which can break hair fibers

Mildly acidic rinses using vinegar (a tablespoon of apple cider vinegar to a quart of water) or lemon juice (a half teaspoon to a quart of water) neutralize alkaline shampoos and make hair shine because acidic substances shrink the hair shaft and encourage the cuticle to lie flat. Curly hair tends to be duller, so more acidic rinses would be necessary. Brunettes can also use coffee (cold or cooled) on their hair. It is slightly acidic, although not as good as lemon juice. An acidic rinse can make curly hair even curlier and straight hair very straight.

Hot water swells the hair shaft and cool water shrinks it and makes hair shiny, so the final rinse after shampooing should be cool as well as mildly acidic.

Porosity

Porosity refers to the ability of a substance to absorb liquids. The porosity of hair is important to its texture. Among other factors, porosity is affected by:

Health	Setting lotions	Climate	Bleaches
Altitude	Dyes	Humidity	Oils
Shampoos	Permanents	Rinses	Straighteners
Conditioners			

To test for porosity, take a small strand of hair and, holding it smooth, run your fingers from the end toward the scalp. If the hair ruffles, it is porous. If wet hair feels spongy when squeezed, takes a long time to dry, and wets very easily, it is unusually porous and vulnerable to damage because the outer protective cuticle is gone and cannot protect the inner shaft of the hair. Porous hair is inelastic and brittle and needs conditioning after every wash, preferably with a low-pH shampoo. Colored hair is often porous. A protein conditioner will help coat each damaged hair shaft, filling in the cracks to shield the hair and retain moisture.

All conditioners add shine and softness, but a protein-enriched conditioner does more: A protein conditioner containing hydrolized animal collagen can stick to the hair shaft and fill in irregularities, cracks, and splits. Although it can do nothing to improve the tensile strength of damaged hair, it can temporarily make the rough hair surface smoother and glossier.

Only conditioners that contain wetting agents (which promote the penetration of water-based solutions into the hair to reduce porosity) and quaternary ammonium salts ("quats") can actually strengthen damaged hair. Check your label to see if a quat is included in your conditioner. These conditioners have a positive electrical charge that facilitates bonding with negatively charged or damaged hair, forming a protective layer on the cuticle that smooths hair. They also decrease the friction between hairs, making combing and brushing less damaging and making hair stronger and more flexible. Deep conditioners left on the hair for twenty or thirty minutes will last through three or four successive shampoos without reapplication.

Here are some conditioners that protect hair:

- Nestlé Balsam Plus Instant Conditioner (Nestlé-Lemur)
- Wella Balsam Instant Conditioner (Wella)
- Breck Basic: Conditioner with Protein (Breck)
- Creme Conditioner de Pantene (Richardson-Vicks)
- Protein Pac Treatment (Vidal Sassoon)
- Infusium 23 Vitamin Hair Treatment (Duart)

Conditioning should be a regular part of your hair-care program. It prevents excess cuticle loss or flyaway hair and helps replenish the natural oils and moisture that give hair flexibility and shine.

Split Ends

Those flyaway, ragged tips of hair that never look quite groomed are an indication that hair keratin is drying and crumbling. Split ends come from the same source as dull hair: repetitive abuse.

Damage to the cuticle leads first to partial splitting of hair fibers, then to splitting of the hair shaft. Cutting off the split ends is a first grooming step (hair should be trimmed every six to eight weeks) but not the solution, because soon the newly trimmed ends will start to fray, too—unless you change your hair habits. Rebuilding the keratin in the entire hair shaft to stop the splitting is not necessary. A program involving both protein conditioners that concentrate on the hair ends and low-pH rinses will help. Don't singe the split ends away—that technique never works.

Preventing Damaged Hair

"Don't do anything to your hair that you wouldn't do to a good sweater." That is good advice, but since you wear your hair every day, you cannot avoid some abuse. At the very least it is wetted, shampooed, dried, and subjected to heat, sun, and cold, all of which are potentially damaging.

Unfortunately, nothing can effectively reverse harm done to hair, because hair is dead tissue, unable to repair itself. A better plan is protection.

Sun and heat break the chemical bonds responsible for hair's strength and deplete cystine, the hair's amino acid and a protein component, leaving hair susceptible to breaking and splitting. Blond or bleached hair, whose melanin (pigment) is missing, is less resistant to weather damage than dark hair, because color is protective. The sun is a particular enemy to smooth texture: It dries and lifts the cuticle around the hair just as it roughens and peels your skin, and the damage is compounded by regular exposure to salt water or the chemically treated water in pools.

Winter cold and winds are no easier on the hair. When the temperature falls below freezing, the moisture in the hair can freeze, too. This expands the shaft and breaks the cuticle, making it unable to protect the inner layers of hair and allowing evaporation of the hair's important moisture. Dry, brittle, damaged hair is the result. (For more on the climate's effect on hair see chapter 7.)

Low-pH Shampoos and Rinses

Low-pH shampoos (with a pH of less than 7 or as announced on the label of the bottle or tube) are slightly acidic and will be milder than high-alkaline shampoos. These shampoos are recommended for chemically treated hair, which is generally more porous. They shrink the hair, making it less absorbent and easier to comb.

Here are two good low-pH commercial rinses:

• New Improved Creme Rinse with Extra Body, pH 3.75 (Breck)
• Aquamarine Conditioning Creme Rinse, pH 3.25 (Revlon)

Shampooing—The Essential of Hair Care

How to Choose the Right Shampoo

To select the shampoo that is best for you read labels carefully. Ingredients are listed in the order of the proportion that is used in the product. The differences between shampoos for dry, normal, and oily hair are based on the types and quantities of detergents and conditioners included in the formulas. Conditioning agents are included in all shampoos; the higher the ratio of detergent to conditioner, the harsher the shampoo (usually one meant for oily hair). For damaged hair, select a shampoo with a high percentage of moisturizers such as wheat germ oil, jojoba oil, lanolin, and panthenol. For dry hair, look for additives such as herbal extract and butyl alcohol.

Here are the ingredients you will see listed on a shampoo label.

- Water is usually listed first.
- Surfactants are the foaming agents.
- Strong detergents, which you can expect to be listed on a shampoo for oily hair, include sodium lauryl sulfate, ammonium lauryl sulfate, and sodium olefin sulfate.
- Mild detergents, best for dry or chemically treated hair, include cocamidopropyl betaine and cocamido betaine.
- Nonionic agents, found in the mildest shampoos, include polysorbate 20, polysorbate 40, sorbitan laurate, sorbitan stearate, and sorbitan palmitate.

Shampooing Damaged Hair

Loving care is necessary for damaged hair. Here are some guidelines:

- Choose a mild shampoo that is formulated for tinted or permanently waved hair, or use baby shampoo. (The same treatment is required for both since the chemicals in the waving process have much the same effect on hair as does overexposure to the sun.) Low-pH shampoos or mild-tar shampoos such as Neutrogena T/Gel are also recommended.
- Shampoo less often and more gently than you usually do. Use only one lathering, and do not allow the lather to remain on your hair for long periods of time.
- Try to keep the shampoo and lather at the scalp to rid the scalp of excess oils and sloughed skin cells. Do not concentrate on shafts or ends of hair.
- Use fingertips, not fingernails, to work in the lather.

Dull hair is not always the result of damaged cuticle. Shampoo residue left on hair can also be dulling (the more ingredients, the more residue may remain), as can overconditioning or using a conditioning shampoo *plus* conditioner. When using conditioner remember that damaged hair absorbs more of it.

Seborrheic Dermatitis (Dandruff)

Dandruff is a very common problem. Stress plays a major role; emotional overload can be a triggering factor in the production of dandruff.

Dandruff appears when epidermal cells turn over at a much faster than normal rate. The dandruff-producing rate is often so rapid that nuclei of the cells can be found in the shed scales (nuclei usually disappear as the normal cell matures). These prematurely matured cells clump together and break away in large dandruff flakes that leave the scalp with fewer top epidermal layers of cells than normal.

In severe cases the eyebrows, eyelashes, ears, and skin behind the ears—even the skin around the nose and on the bridge of the nose—are also involved, and the scaling and redness come with itching, which leads to scratching and a potential infection. Don't mistake the scaling for dry skin— it is just the opposite. Moisturizers won't help and can even make the problem worse.

Dandruff seems to be less prevalent in spring and summer and more prevalent in fall and winter. Dandruff attracts more attention than it deserves when it appears on the shoulders of your dark suits, sweaters, or dresses.

Fighting Flakes

To prevent and treat dandruff, avoid stimulating oil production. Be wary of overbrushing your hair or overmassaging your scalp. While brushing loosens sticky scales, it can stimulate the scalp in the same way that massage will. A simple hairstyle that requires very little manipulation of the hair, and combing with a smooth rubber or shell wide-toothed comb is often all that is needed.

The basic treatment is to clean the scalp with frequent shampooings that rid it of excess scales and possibly slow down the maturation of new cells. Shampooing, like facial cleansing, must be done carefully, and rinsing off all soap and cleanser residues is very important.

Finding the Right Dandruff Shampoo

There are dozens of dandruff shampoos on the market. The most effective products can be grouped by the way they work.

- Those with selenium sulfide or zinc pyrithione work fastest, retarding the cell turnover rate:

Head and Shoulders (Procter & Gamble)	Selsun Blue (Ross)
	Zincon (Lederle)
Selsun (Abbott), by prescription	Sebulon (Westwood)
	Danex (Herbert)

- Those with salicylic acid and sulfur loosen flakes so the flakes can be washed away easily:
  - Sebulex (Westwood) Vanseb (Herbert)
  - X-Seb (Baker/Cummins) Ionil (Owen)

- Those that provide an antibacterial agent reduce the number of bacteria on the scalp and the chance of infections:
  - Betadine Shampoo (Purdue Frederick) Capitrol Cream Shampoo (Westwood), by prescription

- Those with tar retard cell growth:
  - T/Gel (Neutrogena)—the best Polytar (Stiefel)
  - Ionil-T (Owen) Zetar (Dermik)
  - Pentrax (Cooper)

- Some tar shampoos also contain salicylic acid:
  - X-Seb T (Baker/Cummins) Vanseb T (Herbert)

Tar shampoos also have the ability to repair damaged hair (since they are mildly alkaline, they temporarily soften the hair cuticle). Tar shampoos have drawbacks: They can stain blond or silvery hair (although newer products have been improved); some people have irritant and allergic reactions to the tar; and many people can't stand the smell (but this is less of a problem with some of the newer, more "elegant" products). You can always use a regular shampoo afterwards.

Some dandruff shampoos can be drying. To offset this, you can use a mild shampoo for lathering and a dandruff shampoo for the second washing, or alternate between dandruff shampoos and mild ones.

To improve the effectiveness of any medicated shampoo, put a shower cap on after shampoo is lathered on the scalp and leave it on for an hour.

Selenium sulfide and zinc pyrithione shampoos have preventive as well as treatment value and can be used effectively to stave off problems, or they can be used between bouts.

Some of the shampoos listed above use combinations of active ingredients to fight dandruff in the hope that if one ingredient doesn't do the trick then another one will—or that they will work together more effectively than either will work alone.

Buy more than one brand. A common problem with dandruff shampoos is that they work well for some time and then mysteriously stop being effective. Keep switching products. If you don't see any improvement with over-the-counter dandruff shampoos, your dermatologist can prescribe a more effective one.

Recent evidence suggests that yeast may cause seborrheic dermatitis. The antiyeast medication Nizoral-ketoconazole (cream or tablets; Janssen, by prescription) has been used successfully in the treatment of stubborn dandruff.

Using Your Dandruff Shampoo

If your dandruff is severe, you may have thick crusts of scaling skin that should be removed before shampooing so that the shampoo's specially prepared chemicals can be more effective by getting directly to the scalp. You can remove the crusts easily by applying warm mineral oil to the scalp about a half hour before shampooing. Warm the mineral oil by packing a small bottle of it in hot water, and then paint it on the scalp with a wide paintbrush, or use a cotton swab. An alternate treatment is to use P and S liquid (a phenol/saline lotion available from Baker/Cummins), which contains mineral oil and can be applied overnight, then washed off in the morning. Or you can use a bath oil with tar, such as T/Derm Bath Oil (Neutrogena). Wearing a plastic shower cap or a turban made of a warm, wet towel for a few hours will enhance the results.

Shampoo daily:

1. Wet your hair thoroughly and then lather well.
2. Rinse and apply sudsing shampoo again.
3. Using fingertip pads, work the suds into the scalp, stripping it of accumulated grease and cell buildup.
4. Be sure to scrub the hairline and behind your ears. Use a small nail brush or a shampoo brush for this; you want to get all the scales off.
5. Allow the shampoo to remain in contact with the scalp for at least five minutes; this is very important.
6. Rinse and then rinse several times more.

The task is to get your scalp clean while keeping the ends of your hair from being stripped of all their natural oils. Frequent shampooings will not harm your scalp or hair, and using a protein conditioner or a shampoo with a built-in conditioner will help prevent hair from becoming dull and dry. Use a conditioner but only on the ends of the hair; allowing conditioner to rest on your scalp may encourage dandruff. Two recommended new antidandruff conditioning products are T/Gel Scalp Solution and Therapeutic Conditioner (both from Neutrogena).

Setting and Styling—Making Your Hair Part of Your Total Look

Changing your hairstyle might tell the world you have changed your point of view. One of my favorite patients has done just that: When she first came to my office, her golden brown hair was very long and straight; a year later it was short and blond; then it was curly and reddish; now it is shoulder-length and golden once again. Each style had significance: She went from being a law student to being an international banker, and her hairstyle went with her.

Hydrogen/Sulfur Bonds—Hair Shape Determinants

The protein molecules in hair are arranged in organized patterns and held in place by chemical bonds. The way a hair grows from the follicle and its individual shape depend on sulfur and hydrogen. The chemical bonds they form make your hair look like your hair.

To change the shape of your hair, the chemical bonds that keep the hair together must be broken. This can be done by setting and by permanent waving.

The hydrogen bonds can be broken simply by wetting your hair. Each time you wash your hair you break the hydrogen bond; each time you dry your hair you reform it. The perspiration from your scalp when you are jogging can be enough to undo a set and make your hair either droop or frizz.

When hair's hydrogen bonds are broken, it is susceptible to damage. Here is how to protect wet hair:

- After a shower or swim, pat your hair dry rather than rub it.
- Do not stretch or pull your hair until it has dried; if you set it wet, avoid manipulating it too much.
- Finger-comb hair and then comb it with a wide-toothed comb made of plastic or bone. Never use a metal comb or brush—rough surfaces can split the hair fibers and damage the hair cuticle along the entire length of the hair shaft.
- If you use a blow dryer, keep the temperature on low. Hold the nozzle at least six inches from your hair, and move it around frequently. Hair sustains more damage from brushing during blow-drying than from any other type of grooming.

Sulfur bonds are responsible for your hair's strength, elasticity, and solubility. To alter these qualities requires heat or a very strong alkaline solution—the solution used in permanents breaks the sulfur bonds. Excess heat—when straightening or curling hair, for example—can also break sulfur bonds. The result is that hair splits, making it more susceptible to breakage.

Any chemical treatment—permanent waving, straightening, coloring, or bleaching—damages the sulfur bond in hair. If such treatments are undertaken, keep in mind that they may result in more damage. Stick to a home permanent formulated for damaged hair and follow the directions carefully. It takes a long time for broken sulfur bonds to re-form, so don't wash or blow-dry your hair for at least two days after getting a permanent, and keep your hair soft and moist by spraying it often with a mister.

Do not attempt to color and wave your hair at the same time; allow an interval of at least two weeks between the processes. Color first, perm later.

Making Your Hair Stay Put

For stay-put hairstyles, setting lotions, mousses, and gels made of vegetable gums dissolved in water and alcohol have long been used by men and women alike. The water breaks hydrogen bonds within the hair, and the setting or combing re-forms them in new positions. When the water dries, the hair is repositioned and supported by the gums in the gels.

Synthetic polymer resins recently have been incorporated into hair sprays and setting lotions. These plasticizers are more resistant to moisture than gums and so last longer and provide a solution for hard-to-hold and flyaway hair. The drawback is that the plastic film that forms often becomes hard and brittle; it may crack and flake as the hair is combed or moves and that can give the appearance of dandruff.

It is important to use spray products, especially hair sprays, correctly since they can damage the lungs. Most susceptible to lung damage are women with chronic bronchitis, emphysema, or asthma. Direct the nozzle of your aerosol can very carefully and don't breathe in the mist that accompanies even carefully placed applications.

Here are some hair sprays that hold:

- Wella Flex (Wella)
- Final Mist (Clairol)
- Rave (Chesebrough-Pond's)
- Creatif Designing Spray (Redken)

Mousse

Mousses are a new form of setting lotion that can also add temporary color. They work essentially the same as gels, coating the hair to allow it to be sculpted. Mousse is a foam that suspends the lotion with air to make it more manageable, so it can be worked through the hair without drying to a stiff plasticlike coating. Some mousses contain sunscreens, zinc pyrithione (to combat dandruff), or moisturizers (for permed or colored hair).

The best way to apply a mousse is to squirt some on a wide-toothed comb and then comb it through shampooed, towel-dried hair. (Gels are stiffer and work better than mousses on dry hair.) Either let the hair dry naturally or blow-dry it. Some recommended new products are:

- Chocolate Mousse—also Strawberry and Lemon (Zotos)
- Sophisticated Look (Revlon)
- Natural Henna—also Walnut (Klorane)
- Vidal Sassoon Mousse (Vidal Sassoon)
- Valence Styling Mousse (L'Oréal)

For highlights or a change in shading, apply color mousse all over the hair (highlights) or on different portions of the hair. A darker shade on the sides makes the hair look longer. Color mousses will not totally cover gray hair, but they do make it blend in while providing highlights.

If you are caught in the rain with a color mousse you could drip color. To prevent this color runoff use hair spray after the mousse has dried.

A note on hair holders: A brisk brushing or combing changes the hair's electrical charge and uncontrollable flyaway hair is the result. To prevent static electricity, avoid tight-bristled brushes and overbrushing. Use fingers and hands to style and smooth the hair, or choose a wide-toothed antistatic comb or brush. (I have found that Tek, a brand made in Italy, works well.)

Color Problems

The sun has a bleaching effect on hair. While some people like the streaked effect of sun bleaching, others do not. Tinting the hair to even out the streaks is risky, but a certain amount of camouflage can be provided by temporary water-soluble color rinses. Since these preparations do not penetrate hair shafts, they can do no damage. If the result is not to your liking you can simply shampoo it away. To help prevent sun discolorations, use conditioners and styling products with sunscreen added—such as Revlon's Flex Sun and Sport System or Pantene's Sunbrella Stylers.

Gray Hair

The color of hair is due to the melanin granules in the cortex of the hair shaft. When, usually through age, the number of melanocytes in a hair bulb diminishes and melanin production decreases, then stops, the hair turns white. As more and more of these white hairs mix with the naturally pigmented hair, a gray effect is produced. True gray hairs are actually very rare. Dark hair doesn't gray earlier than blond hair, it just seems to because of the sharper contrast. Graying usually starts at about age thirty and continues for thirty years, until the seventh decade of life, when hair often becomes completely white. For reasons not completely understood, gray hair tends to be thicker than pigmented hair.

Worry does not turn hair gray. No one really knows why at a certain time the production of melanin stops. Heredity is certainly a factor, since certain families gray early and others late. Sometimes, for reasons not completely understood, exhaustion or a severe shock that saddens life does seem to contribute to graying. But hair on the head cannot turn gray overnight, because its color was formed months or even years earlier. Pigment production can stop suddenly, so that new hair growth is white.

Gray hair sometimes takes on a yellowish tinge. To prevent this, avoid dandruff shampoos containing selenium sulfide or chloroxine, setting lotions, tar shampoos, cigarette smoke, and chemotherapeutic agents.

The easiest way to get rid of the yellowish tinge is to use a blue rinse: Add a teaspoon of laundry bluing to the clear water in your bathroom sink as a final rinse; allow it to remain on your hair for about ten minutes, then rinse it away.

Diet and Hair Color

From time to time various diets have been touted to prevent the graying of hair: Diets high in vitamin B, including a lot of grape juice, or rich in some other nutrient have been tried. No one has proved that they work.

Deficiencies of copper and zinc (minerals found largely in fruits, vegetables, and whole grains) have been implicated in some cases of premature graying. A folic acid deficiency may also cause premature graying—women on estrogen-dominant oral contraceptives run a greater risk of folic acid deficiency. Taking supplements of copper and zinc or folic acid will help only those women who actually suffer a deficiency. It will have no effect on other women.

Once hair grays, little can be done except make the gray look as attractive as possible—or color the hair artificially.

Diet and Hair Growth

Since nutrients are needed for hair growth, diet can affect the rate of growth and texture of hair. The B vitamins accelerate protein synthesis in the hair follicles and include folic acid. Brewer's yeast is a source of B complex vitamins. Vitamin C is necessary for effective absorption of folic acid. Iron and zinc are also needed for healthy hair. Be sure your diet also includes:

- Protein—obtained from fish, fowl, lean meats, eggs, beans, nuts, dairy products
- Niacin—obtained from chicken, peanuts, wheat germ, milk, legumes, lean beef, mushrooms
- Vitamin B_6 (pyridoxine)—obtained from wheat germ, cereals, liver, meat, eggs, bananas, milk, potatoes, lima beans
- Vitamin B_{12}—obtained from liver, meat, eggs, milk
- Vitamin A—obtained from yellow vegetables, liver, liver oils

For more information on diet, refer to chapter 17.

Hair Analysis for Determining Dietary Imbalance

The use of hair analysis as a basis for medical diagnoses has been discussed in magazine articles in recent years, but its reliability has not been scientifically substantiated. Calculating mineral excesses and deficiencies in the hair should not be used to evaluate general health because the mineral content of hair is not indicative of present nutritional status. For example, a mineral may be found in a normal or high quantity in the hair while there is a deficiency in the body. (It's also possible to get different reports from the same sample.) Furthermore, normal ranges of hair minerals have not been established and hair has no vitamins. However, hair analysis can determine whether or not a person has been exposed to toxic levels of a metal or mineral.

To the extent that hair analysis is reliable, it is so only when done under carefully controlled conditions and supported by other methods of trace metal analysis.

Some salons as well as special hair-analysis laboratories use computers to assess your hair's condition. Shampoos with selenium, hair color with lead, bleaches, and pollution may actually affect the tests more than diet does. To determine dietary deficiencies, see your physician and learn more about your personal nutritional needs.

Hair-Care Check Chart

Match hair texture, care, and styling.

Texture	Shampoo	Conditioner	Styling
Dry hair: dry, brittle, dull, split ends	Mild/baby shampoo 1 lathering only	Deep conditioner with emollients	Avoid rollers. Avoid dryers.
Oily hair: greasy one day after shampooing	Cleansing shampoos 2 latherings Allow shampoo to remain on scalp.	Oil-free conditioner Avoid deep conditioners.	Avoid hats.
Combination hair: oily roots, dry ends	Use 2 shampoos—gentle, then normal.	Condition dry ends only.	
Fine hair: lacks body, will not hold set, static electricity	Very mild shampoo 1 lathering only	Use instant conditioners.	Color hair to add body. Use thickeners and styling gels.
Damaged hair: breaks easily, dry and brittle when combed	Low-pH shampoo	Deep conditioners	Tug-free style

---

A Hairy Tale

I recall a sequence in a movie that showed a woman leaving a salon to rush home and wash her hair—because she hated what they did to her. I've had that experience, and it *is* awful. Before you "give your hair" to anyone, know what you want and make sure your hairdresser knows, too.

14

HOW TO HAVE

FAT HAIR,

AND LOTS OF IT

I often notice a patient's thinning hair when I am treating her for other skin conditions. Or a patient brings up her concern by asking me, "What do you do with your hair? It is so thick." (I have my parents to thank for that—hair thickness, like many other characteristics, is inherited.)

Completely bald women are a rarity, but thinning hair is a common problem; most women suffer some hair loss during their lives. Because our society places such high premium on thick, full hair, the experience is very distressing.

It is not unusual for a middle-aged woman to seek help for wrinkles or skin discolorations yet assume that thinning hair is inevitable. It isn't.

What happens to all that thick hair of childhood?

Abnormal hair loss has a wide variety of possible causes. Dermatologists, who regularly treat hair problems and alopecia (the medical term for balding), can evaluate your scalp's and hair's condition and suggest probable causes after taking a family and personal history.

A woman's hair loss can be the result of perfectly natural genetic factors, as with men who are genetically programmed for baldness. Or it may be the result of any number of different conditions, many of which can be corrected.

Why Hair Thins and What Can Be Done

Cosmetic Alopecia

Waving, coloring, bleaching, straightening, and other processes use chemicals that can damage the hair even when they are correctly applied. If a procedure is used too often, solutions are left on too long, or two procedures are tried closely together, your hair may be damaged, start breaking, and leave thin or even bald areas.

Excessive or improper shampooing, brushing, and combing can also cause problems. Constant teasing, tight curling, braiding, dragging a brush across the scalp, pulling with an elastic, or the frequent use of a rough comb that tears away a few hairs each time it passes through the hair can all produce thinning.

Hair help: To stop or reduce this thinning, be more careful. Treat your hair as the precious and delicate adornment it is.

Alopecia Areata

This type of balding usually appears in small circular patches about the size of a coin. However, in severe cases it can lead to the loss of all the hair on the scalp (alopecia totalis) and sometimes all body hair (alopecia universalis), even eyebrows and lashes. Some 10 to 20 percent of those who suffer this also experience changes in their nails, such as numerous little pits in the nail surface (often in horizontal or vertical rows), thickening, roughness, ridging, and brittleness.

No age group is free of risk; the cause of the condition is unknown—many women affected by alopecia areata are in excellent health.

It is known that alopecia areata is more common in those whose blood relatives have had it. In other cases it is stress-induced. Acute stress (an accident, for example) is a common precursor of alopecia areata. There is excessive hair loss before clearly defined round patches are visible. The more extensive the condition, the more difficult it is to cure. Alopecia areata has a tendency to recur.

Hair help: In some cases, the hair regrows spontaneously. In different circumstances, repeated applications of an allergen-irritant by a dermatologist to produce contact dermatitis is used to induce hair regrowth. That works in more than half the women treated, but the therapy must be continued for several months. Topical, intralesional, or systemic steroids are also used successfully.

Postpartum Alopecia

In the first two or three months after giving birth, some women are shocked to notice large quantities of hair in their combs and brushes. This increase in shedding lasts from a few months to a year. It is actually the result of hair being in a prolonged growth stage during pregnancy. (For more about this kind of thinning, see chapter 21.)

Hair help: After the resting hair is shed and once your natural hormone balance is restored, your hair will return to its normal thickness.

Fever Alopecia

It is not completely understood why hair is sometimes affected by high fever, but from six weeks to three months after having a fever higher than 103°F, such as with a severe infection or flu, a woman may be bothered by some hair thinning. This is probably caused by protein depletion.

Hair help: Fever loss usually reverses itself. To speed up recovery, topical steroid lotions or intralesional steroids can be used.

Drug Alopecia

A small percentage of people taking certain prescription and nonprescription drugs for other medical problems may experience some temporary and reversible thinning. Drugs known to have these occasional side effects include:

- Heparin and other blood thinners
- Antiarthritic drugs
- Some antidepressants and amphetamines
- Beta blockers (for heart problems and high blood pressure)
- Some antibiotics
- Chemotherapeutic agents
- Antiulcer drugs
- Lithium
- Gold
- Some thyroid medications
- Cholesterol-lowering agents
- Aspirin, over long-term use
- Vitamin A derivatives (e.g., Accutane)
- Cough medicines containing iodides
- Lead salts or arsenic salts
- Boric acid (found in mouthwash)

A few drugs used in cancer treatment will cause the cells of the hair to stop dividing; hair shafts then become thin and break off as they emerge from the scalp.

Hair help: Most patients regrow their hair after their treatment ends.

Surgery Alopecia

Major surgery is a tremendous shock to the system. Within two or three months after surgery, many recuperating patients notice signs of hair loss, probably due to anesthesia. Bypass surgery for obesity causes crash diet alopecia (see below).

Hair help: This usually reverses itself within a few months.

Anemia Alopecia

A low level of iron has been linked to the thinning of hair in some women. The deficiency can be detected by laboratory tests. Women who experience heavy periods and have dry and brittle hair and excessive hair loss should be checked for blood iron levels.

Hair help: Women, particularly after giving birth, should be sure their diet contains sufficient iron. The problem can also be corrected by taking ferrous sulfate or other iron supplements. (For more about hair growth and diet, see chapter 13.)

Crash Diet Alopecia

Whether because of the hormonal readjustments they provoke or for other reasons such as lack of protein, certain crash diets—those involving the loss of twenty-five pounds or more in a month—can result in hair loss. Vegetarians and anorexics who develop protein malnutrition also sometimes suffer hair loss because, in order to conserve protein, their bodies shift nutrients from growing hair to more important functions. This alopecia usually appears all over the scalp about three months after crash dieting begins.

Hair help: Eating a properly balanced diet is the key to reversing this condition. (For more about the need for an adequate diet, see chapter 17.)

Thyroid Gland Alopecia

Both excessive and insufficient activity of the thyroid gland can cause hair loss. Fragile hair and partial loss of eyebrows usually indicates hypothyroidism. (Poor kidney and/or liver function may also result in alopecia.)

Hair help: Conditions such as this can be diagnosed, and with proper treatment of the underlying causes the thinning of the hair can be reversed.

Birth Control Alopecia

Oral contraceptives contain synthetic estrogens and synthetic progestin. If you are predisposed to thinning hair, thinning may be accelerated by the effects produced by androgen-dominant contraceptives. Sometimes hair loss may begin after stoppage of estrogen-dominant oral contraceptives. The causes are the same as for postpartum alopecia (see above).

Hair help: Birth control alopecia usually reverses within six months.

Familial Alopecia

If your male or female relatives suffer from thinning hair, you may be prone to the problem as well. The trait can be inherited from either side of the family. Its signs are observable by the time you are twenty, and often even earlier. This form of alopecia usually begins gradually and is localized at the top of the head.

Hair help: None of us can change who our parents are—few would want to. Thinning hair may run in your family, but some really wonderful attributes and talents probably do, too. Hair will not grow back by itself. Treatment with minoxidil, discussed later in this chapter, is an option.

Seborrhea

Untreated seborrheic dermatitis is a common cause of hair loss in women. This can be prevented or reversed if the scalp problem is kept under control.

Hair help: This condition is not easy to control—but with care, it can be done. (For more about hair care and a remedial program see chapter 13.)

Other Causes of Hair Loss

Alopecia can also be brought on by vitamin formulations containing iodides and high doses of vitamins A and E and selenium. If the condition is the result of exposure to radiation, it is most likely permanent. Typically, alopecia also occurs in the late stages of syphilis.

Stress can cause a large number of hair follicles to go into a resting stage simultaneously. The onset is usually very sudden and occurs several months after the stressful event. Fortunately, as stress decreases, hair grows back, although it is usually lighter and thinner at first.

Some forms of hair loss are followed by spontaneous regrowth; other types can be treated by a dermatologist. A consultation with a dermatologist may be necessary, if only for your peace of mind.

Hair Transplants

When a woman loses her hair permanently, for whatever reason, it follows, as the night the day, that she will strongly desire to replace it. This intense and predictable demand has given rise to countless folk remedies, few if any of which work, and to surgical techniques, which usually do work.

Hair transplants are used most often for irreversible androgenic alopecia, when an inherited predisposition forces hair follicles to convert to the resting stage prematurely under the influence of male hormones. Hair transplants have been greatly improved in recent years and can be a permanent solution to baldness. The transplants are round plugs of hair-bearing scalp tissue moved from one area of the head—usually the back of the head—to another to selectively redistribute hair over the entire scalp. (The hair on the back of the head has to be quite thick, and this is more common in men than in women.) Hair transplants do not give you more hair, just a better distribution that allows you to select a more flattering hairstyle and makes your hair seem thicker.

The improvements are not immediate: To prevent severe disappointment, I always forewarn my patients that transplanted hair usually falls out very soon after the procedure (two to eight weeks later) but will regrow several months later. It is also possible for *non*transplanted hair to fall out temporarily as a result of surgical trauma.

The Transplant Procedure and Subsequent Hair Growth

Although the idea of transplanting hair is an ancient one, the hair-grafting technique used most widely today was developed in 1959 by Norman Orentreich, M.D. The procedure is usually done under local anesthesia in a doctor's office. The hair grafts are taken with a punch, an instrument similar to a small cookie cutter. The "plugs" are inserted into a recipient space just a tiny bit smaller than the plug, ensuring a very snug fit and helping to secure it. The grafts are spaced far enough apart so that nourishment from surrounding blood vessels is sufficient to ensure the survival of each plug. Time must elapse before another set of grafts is placed into the intervening spaces in order to allow blood vessels the chance to provide enough nourishment.

After transplantation the grafts form crusts that are shed—along with the hair shafts protruding from the tissue—within three to four weeks following the procedure. New hairs begin to grow about eight weeks after the grafts are placed. Therefore, a minimum of ten to twelve weeks must pass after each transplant session before new hair growth becomes visible.

Up to 100 small plugs of hair can be transplanted in one session at the dermatologist's office. Many sessions are required to fill in a large thin area. The sessions are usually scheduled with at least four-week intervals.

Hair transplants are not for the impatient—they can't bring immediate gratification. But they can make a world of difference if you have a localized thin area that makes you feel uncomfortable and you are ready to wait for the results.

Contraindications to hair transplants include a history of bleeding disorders, healing problems, high blood pressure, and a tendency to scar formation.

Patients may experience some minor discomfort while the dermatologist works, but the insertion of plugs is done with the help of a local anesthetic, so the procedure itself is relatively painless. Bleeding is seldom a problem; any that occurs is easily controlled with pressure or a small stitch. The patient leaves the office with a bandage to be removed within twenty-four hours. Perhaps best of all, the procedure works; the acceptance rate is excellent. For a week after the procedure the patient should avoid vigorous exercise and sun exposure, which can discolor healing areas.

Hair usually grows at the rate of one-half inch a month, so a wait of six to eight months is necessary before any real improvement can be seen. Final results may take as long as a year. During that time, special techniques of hair styling and grooming may be used to encourage the new growth and hide the signs of the recent surgery. What makes the trouble and waiting worthwhile is that the transplants will last a lifetime.

Although the procedure described here is used most often on men—because far more men than women go bald—transplants work even better on women. Their long (though thinning) hair near the transplant site can more easily be styled to disguise the transplants. Also, in balding women the hairline is usually preserved. Once new hair starts growing in the transplanted tissue, the transplants themselves become virtually invisible. Perming and/or coloring helps blend it in.

An Anti-Baldness Drug?

Minoxidil (Loniten is its brand name), a drug from Upjohn used since the late 1970s to treat some hypertensive patients, has been found to have the side-effect of stimulating hair growth. It has recently been used as a topical medication in the treatment of balding, with wonderful results. In various clinical tests, solutions of 1 to 5 percent were applied to the scalp of patients with androgenic alopecia and 20 to 25 percent of them showed some improvement, including new hair growth.

Minoxidil retards hair loss in almost everyone. It also often restores hair color within a few months of application; however, the color is lost when medication is stopped. Until a minoxidil solution specifically for scalp treatment is approved by the FDA, it is important that any minoxidil solution intended for the treatment of balding be prepared by a pharmacist who is familiar with it.

In patients who respond, regrowth usually begins four to six months after treatment is started. But application of the minoxidil solution must be continued indefinitely to keep the regrown hair.

It is impossible to predict who will respond, but the following factors appear to improve one's chances:

- Thinning has occurred within the last few years.
- The balding area is small (less than 10 centimeters in diameter).
- There are numerous fine hairs in the area.
- The patient is relatively young.

Minoxidil treatment seems to work better on women with male-pattern baldness than on men. It has also been used in conjunction with hair transplants to increase hair density and prevent further loss.

The mechanism of hair regrowth following minoxidil application is not yet completely understood. The drug most likely increases blood supply to the skin and so enlarges hair follicles. It can also change hair thickness and color, and it probably interferes with aging of the follicle, too. The baldness-treatment formulation, to be called Regaine, is awaiting FDA approval for topical use. Although not 100 percent effective, minoxidil has promise and is relatively safe. Hope springs eternal, and occasionally hope proves to have been justified.

In the West a woman's hair has traditionally been highly prized. In ancient Egypt and Rome wigs were used to hide baldness. Today we look to medicine for a cure. As medicine advances, so does our need for it, for alopecia is on the increase, perhaps because of the prevalence of fad diets and the ever-increasing stresses of modern life.

15

COLOR AND CURL! CHANGE YOUR HAIR TO CHANGE YOUR LIFE

If you don't like your natural hair color, change it. No other cosmetic improvement is as fast and satisfying. I often change the color of my hair and feel more natural in my new color than with the natural one. More than 34 million American women a year who use rinses, dyes, and other hair-coloring products appear to share this philosophy.

Hair Coloring—What's It All About?

Hair coloring involves the addition of an artificial color to natural hair pigments. Hair lightening, in contrast, is the removal of color from naturally pigmented hair. Skill in coloring your own hair is both an art and a science. New products are constantly being created to take some of the guesswork out of hair coloring, but a good deal of mystery remains.

Before dyeing your hair a new color, look closely at the color of your natural hair—the matter isn't as simple as it sounds. An apparently uniform dark blond to medium brown head of hair proves to be made up of a combination of black, red, and blond strands. Different hairs from the same scalp may range from warm golden brown to mousy murky brown.

The dull hair that frequently troubles blondes and brunettes in their forties and fifties seems faded mostly because brightly colored hairs are mixed with gray hairs. Gray or white hairs mixed with black hair are more distinctly visible, giving a dramatic salt-and-pepper effect rather than the effect of dullness. I sometimes encourage gray-haired friends and patients to stay gray. Some of them have returned to gray after years of dyeing and love it.

Temporary Colors

Rinse in; wash away. Hair rinses cover the hair shaft, disguising its natural pigments. Visualize a brown piece of paper, then imagine covering it with a film of red plastic; the color turns to a glowing, shining auburn. The color deposited by a rinse remains on the hair only until the next shampoo, which can be either an advantage or a disadvantage.

I've often used a rinse just to see what a new color might look like. Rinses are harmless. They also:

- Are the easiest of all hair colorings for home use
- Intensify your own hair color
- Add highlights by coloring strands in a slightly lighter color
- Are inexpensive, excellent temporary camouflages for gray hair
- Coat the hair shaft, making it slightly thicker, and so add body to thin hair
- Are forgiving—mistakes are easily washed away

If you don't expect too much from a temporary hair color or rinse, you'll not be disappointed. Dramatic changes are beyond their powers, for they do not contain much pigment. If they contained more, it would come off on your scalp rather than stay on your hair. (Actually, some pigment may come off when you're involved in active sports or you wear a warm hat and your scalp perspires heavily.)

When choosing your first rinse, try a shade that is slightly darker and richer than your natural color. Use the product sparingly until you get to know it. Although rinses wash out easily, some can dull the natural shine of your hair by leaving a gummy coating on the hair shaft. Also beware of using rinses on damaged hair. When the outer layer of a hair (the cuticle) has been damaged, the hair is porous and will absorb more color than its healthy neighbors. If a great many of your hairs are damaged, the coloring that results from a rinse may be uneven. Here are some hair rinses that work well for many women:

- Picture Perfect Color Rinse (Clairol)
- Fanci-Full Rinse (Roux)
- Protein Color Rinse (Nestlé)

Quick Color Fix

Crayons, color sticks, and color brushes are available in many shades. They are compounded with soaps or synthetic waxes and coat the hair very much the way mascara coats your eyelashes. These products are for touching up areas where new growth is beginning to show and should be used only between shampoos or major colorings.

Be careful to avoid getting any color on the scalp as you strive to color individual hairs just where they emerge. Because these colors are so waxy they can irritate the scalp or sensitize it, leading to itching and even secondary infection from scratching. I'm not really sold on these temporary touch-ups. I've seen them misused too often, and unless they are artfully applied they look messy and strange.

Some hair-color creams and color sprays are used for theatrical effects. Use them seldom if ever, and wash them away immediately. They don't always come off easily.

Semipermanent Colors

Modern semipermanent dyes no longer contain peroxide, ammonia, or other chemicals likely to destroy hair shaft cuticles; they are alkaline and lift the cuticle, allowing some color change to take place. They can still cause an allergic reaction, so it is important to follow the manufacturer's directions carefully and to try a patch test before applying the product to all of your hair. Semipermanent color enhances or enriches your own natural color. Most of these tinting products contain built-in conditioners to protect your hair while processing it. Be sure to use an acidic (low-pH) shampoo after using any tinting product, to reduce its damaging effect.

Some of the newer products not only coat the hair but have a low (5 percent) penetration of the hair shaft for more lasting results. One application can cover gray, take away a faded, too-much-sun look, and generally rev up the tone of your natural color. However, they are often thin and watery to apply and have an unfortunate tendency to run down the face and neck. Available products include:

- Excellence Extra Rich Hair Color (L'Oréal)
- Preference (L'Oréal)
- Nice'n Easy (Clairol)
- Clairesse (Clairol)

Most of the semipermanent hair colors are formulated to last four to six weeks, but in actual practice how long the color lasts depends on the number of times you shampoo.

Permanent Colors

These colors become part of the hair shaft. To be rid of them, they must be grown out because, although they fade, they don't wash away completely. Three kinds of dyes are used: vegetable, metallic, and aniline dyes.

Vegetable Dyes

The most popular of the vegetable dyes is henna, a red-orange tint that can build up on the hair to give it body and added shine. It looks good on brown hair but unfortunately doesn't cover gray well. Made from the dried leaves of the *Lawsonia spinosa* or *Lawsonia alba* plant that grows in Asia and the Near East, it can be very messy to apply, stains everything it touches, dries and stiffens the hair (for this reason, it is good for oily hair). Once you henna your hair, very little else can be done with it until it grows out. Because henna builds up on the hair shaft, it shouldn't be used more than three times a year. The color doesn't allow for permanent waving, straightening, or coloring with semipermanent dyes. A popular brand of henna is Avigal (distributed by Avigal, N.Y.).

Chamomile has also been used as a dye. It functions more like a bleach than a dye, brightening and lightening more than changing color.

It's easy to color your hair with chamomile:

1. Use three to five chamomile tea bags (available at many health food stores).
2. Steep the bags until you have about a quart of tea; allow to cool.
3. Open the bags and apply the wet leaves to the area of the hair you want to color; then cover the leaves with a plastic cap.
4. Allow the leaves to remain on the hair for about fifteen minutes.
5. Rinse the leaves away with water, then rinse the hair with the cooled tea.

The French believe chamomile has beneficial effects for the skin and hair.

As a rule, vegetable hair dyes are quite safe and probably are not absorbed.

Metallic Dyes

Metallic dyes and compound dyes are never used professionally, because they leave hair dull, devoid of highlights, and generally harsh and brittle to the touch. As they fade they sometimes leave the hair with grotesque colors varying from greenish to purplish. To keep these colors looking fresh, more dye must be applied every day. These dyes are the basis of many "gradual coloring" products regularly sold to men to "restore" gray hair to a youthful shade. Metallic dyes must be removed before coloring hair with any other product is attempted. Allergic reactions to metallic dyes are extremely rare.

Aniline Dyes

Most modern hair colors are based on aniline (synthetic) dyes that work by mixing a dye with a developer. At first the dye molecules are small and able to penetrate the hair shaft's cuticle; once inside they begin to react with the oxygen of the developer (hydrogen peroxide). A chemical reaction takes place and the cortex of the hair is colored. Because the molecules of the dye are now swollen they cannot get back through the cuticle. Shampooing cannot dislodge them. The hair shaft is permanently colored.

Because many people are allergic to aniline dyes, every product on the market includes directions for a patch test to take before the dye is used. The test is essential and should not be skipped. At the first sign of any redness or irritation, stop using the dye.

If you have a reaction to a dye, you may be reacting to a particular color, not to aniline dyes as such; try a new shade before rejecting the project. If you are reacting to a home coloring kit, try having your hair colored professionally—the formula is different and you may avoid a reaction. Aniline dyes can be absorbed through the skin.

Never use aniline dyes anywhere around the eyes. If you have any allergy or even sensitivity to the products, your eyes can be in danger. FDA regulations forbid any eyelash or eyebrow product to contain aniline dyes.

Bleaching

Tinting or dyeing hair to a darker shade can be fairly easy because of the number of products available and the creativity of chemists. Lightening colors, or blonding, is somewhat more complex, requiring two steps, or a "double process." (The Cosmetic, Toiletry and Fragrance Association warns that a limited amount of hair dye is absorbed by the user. Over a period of several years that amount can add up. Bleaches have no coloring agents.)

1. Stripping and Prelightening

To lighten hair, it must first be prelightened—that is, stripped of its natural color—and then colored with a mild dye to the desired shade. Among available creams, oils, and powder bleaches, cream lighteners are the most popular and hydrogen peroxide is most often the active ingredient. To speed the liberation of oxygen in peroxide and dissolution of melanin, ammonia or another alkaline substance such as sodium peroxide is added. The hydrogen peroxide solution damages the cuticle of the hair shaft, allowing the bleach to penetrate the hair's cortex and lighten the coloring pigment there. When hair is bleached some of its proteins break down and the hair loses some of its tensile properties; the hair becomes vulnerable to breakage and dryness and must be treated with great care. Avoid overbleaching (bleach should only be applied to regrown hair, not to hair that has already been bleached).

White or gray hair also requires a certain amount of prelighting to make it porous enough to receive the coloring agent or toner. Since white or gray has very little color, very little bleaching is required—just enough to open the cuticle and allow the new color to penetrate. Red hair is difficult to bleach because its pigment is resistant to bleaching. Sometimes bleaching red hair will just make it redder.

2. Dyeing

Once the hair is bleached, it must be dyed to the right shade. That means further penetration and insertion of color into the hair's cortex. (That is why the procedure is called double process dyeing.) If you don't want a yellow tint or bleached hair, a diluted blue dye rinse will help.

These rounds of chemical and mechanical manipulation make hair very porous and weak. Color fillers such as color mousses or color conditioners may be used to help repair the damage. A filler is a jellylike substance made of protein that tends to even out the porosity along the entire shaft of the hair. This makes the hair reflect light evenly and shine more.

I am often asked how I keep my hair so shiny. I do it by being careful: I am careful not to dye often, I am careful never to do two processes at the same time, and I am careful to go only to a color professional I trust completely. I would much rather have too little color than lose or damage my hair.

Streaking and Frosting

Lightening selected strands of hair has many advantages. It can create a more natural look than a flat overall color, since most hair, especially light-colored hair, is affected by oxidation and naturally has lighter streaks in it already. The procedure can also be used to highlight certain sections of the face by creating a halo effect. The major benefit of such selective lightening is perhaps that it prevents a harsh line of demarcation between newly colored and natural hair, so roots are never as obvious.

Allergic Reactions to Hair Dyes

Although most drugstore hair dyes can be used by most women, they still pose occasional allergy problems. The most dangerous hair coloring ingredients are the coal tar and petroleum dyes. Although they are more common in permanent dyes, they can still be found in older products sold as ordinary dyes. If you develop a reaction—a rash or a burning sensation involving the scalp, and perhaps the ears, eyelids, fingertips, hands, neck, or swelling of the entire face (usually a few hours or a day after the application of any home-use dye)—switch brands or locate a professional supply house and ask for a product with the same color but formulated in a different way. Any slight scalp irritation can be treated with a mild nonprescription hydrocortisone lotion. It should clear up in three to five days. If it doesn't, see your dermatologist.

Paraphenylenediamine, a chemical in many synthetic permanent hair dyes, causes many women to have allergic reactions, most frequently middle-aged women. The compound is very similar to a chemical used in PABA sunscreens, so if you are allergic to those sunscreens, or to sulfa and topical anesthetics such as benzocaine or procaine, you may suffer the same reaction to hair dyes. To minimize the chances of a problem, do a patch test before each application of a dye. Sensitivity to a product can appear at any time, even if you have used the product before. If you know you have this allergy, you can safely use Colorific Color Style 'n Gel (Vidal Sassoon).

The Safety of Hair Dyes

As a dermatologist, I am often asked about hair dye safety, especially by pregnant women and those in their childbearing years. As a woman who dyes her hair, I, too, am concerned. The question of safety has to do with the absorption of hair dyes. However, in studies to date, animals have not developed cancers or other abnormalities after their skin and fur were painted with hair dyes.

Here is what is known about dye absorption:

- Aniline dyes are absorbed by penetration through the skin.
- Vegetable dyes are probably not absorbed.
- Bleaches are probably not absorbed.
- Metallic dyes are minimally absorbed.

Although we do not know what the dangers are, whenever a chemical is absorbed, a risk is being taken.

Always use plastic or rubber gloves when applying dye to hair. Your nails, like your hair, are made of keratin and can pick up the color of the dye, as can the horny layer of the skin on your hands. Follow the directions on the manufacturer's inserts *exactly*. Too much caution is hardly possible. Avoid getting the slightest spatter into your eyes. If dye does get into your eyes, wash it out immediately with plain lukewarm water. If irritation persists, consult your doctor.

Color Care Conditioners

Color-treated hair needs special conditioners and very gentle cleansing. Always use products specially designed for colored hair. Once hair has been colored, its cuticle layer has been lifted or altered, and the hair shaft is roughened. Rinses and conditioners should become an important part of your hair treatment routine.

Conditioners are designed to coat and give body to damaged hair. They are usually creams or liquids. Most contain lanolin, moisturizers, oils, and proteins in combination. Most conditioners are meant to be applied to damp, freshly shampooed hair. Stay away from cream rinses that promise to leave your hair tangle-free—these usually include small quantities of ammonium salts, which can weaken dyed hair. If you have used an aniline dye, avoid rinses that are based on natural or herbal dyes, because they will build up and tinge the hair color.

Timed Conditioners

Best for dry or slightly damaged hair, timed conditioners are applied to hair, allowed to remain on one to five minutes, and then rinsed out. The hair is then styled and set. Most such products are based on the fact that an acidic coating will reduce the damaging effect of coloring and bleaching. These conditioners tighten the cuticle and then coat the hair shaft with oil. When a conditioner is marked as neutralizing, it has a low pH; it is intended to prevent hair damage and, more importantly, to alleviate scalp irritation from the alkaline solutions of hair dyes.

Styling Conditioners

Best for healthy hair, styling conditioners (balsam conditioners are an example) are often resin based. They coat the hair shaft and keep the hair soft by keeping it moist. They also add to the thickness of individual hairs, helping to keep them manageable.

Penetrating Conditioners

Best for chemically damaged or sun-dried hair, penetrating conditioners utilize hydrolized protein, which consists of tiny fragments of protein able to pass through the cuticle layer of the hair and penetrate its cortex. These conditioners will replace some of the damaged keratin of the hair. They improve texture, equalize porosity, and increase hair elasticity. However, if the excess isn't rinsed away, the hair can be left gummy and eventually will weaken.

Problems Associated with Dyed Hair

Dyed hair, like any other, can be host to flakes of dandruff. Avoid harsh alkaline shampoos. Also avoid tar-based dandruff shampoos, especially if your hair is lightened. The tar in these shampoos can be discoloring, as are the selenium sulfide and chloroxine. The least damaging antidandruff products contain zinc pyrithione. Although they are alkaline, you can offset them by using an acid rinse right after shampooing.

If you want to straighten your hair or get a permanent, remember that dyed hair is often dry and brittle. To minimize the chance of further damaging the natural bond that holds your hair together, wait several weeks after coloring before having your hair permed.

Some Precautions to Take with Dyed Hair

- Dyed hair is very easily damaged by the sun. The sun's dehydrating heat can break the keratin fibers in hair and leave you with broken or split ends. Wear a sun hat—it's better for your face, too.
- Avoid swimming in chlorinated pools, as chlorine is sure to damage your hair further. If you do swim, wear a cap.
- Cold and wind are destructive. Hair dyes weaken the cuticle layer of each hair; without this shielding, moisture evaporates more rapidly from your hair, making wintry blasts lethal to it. Keep your hair covered in cold or windy weather.

Permanents and Hair Straightening

The permanent wave as we know it today is an invention of this century, although combinations of water, heat, and borax were used in earlier centuries to break the normal bonds that control the hair and then re-form it into either curlier or straighter tresses. The acid permanent, known since 1970, requires heat.

Home permanent waves (known since 1941) depend on chemicals, not heat, but their use constitutes a violent attack on the normal structure of the hair shaft, actually changing the keratin fibers of the hair. Permanent waving solutions can dissolve hair in the same way a chemical depilatory does; timing is vital to their success. The time, the way the hair is rolled, and the strength of the chemicals used make the difference between a tight perm, a soft perm, and a body perm. A properly done permanent can make hair look fuller and thicker.

Straightening Solutions

Body wave perms are mild softenings designed to give only a small amount of curl to the hair so that it has more volume. Straightening solutions are very similar to permanent waving solutions and often also use thioglycolate compounds to attack and soften the hair and break its natural bonds. Larger perm rods are used. The difference is that the hair is re-formed to be straight, not curly. As with permanent waving, straightening solutions should not be used more than three or four times a year. The body wave lasts up to four months.

Evaluating Permanents

Permanent waving is an art as well as a science. The home kit user, just as much as the professional, must evaluate dozens of factors: timing, type, and concentration of solutions to be used, the condition of the hair and scalp, and more. Here are some factors that can't be ignored, if you want a successful permanent and undamaged hair.

Length of the hair. Waves seem to work best on hair that is twelve to eighteen inches long. If too short, the hair kinks because it gets too much solution and is wound too tightly. If too long, the hair nearest the scalp gets curled more than the ends because the rollers cannot provide equal tension over the full length of the hair. The weight of long hair will in any event soon naturally straighten the curls and defeat the purpose of a permanent.

Porosity of the hair. Porosity determines the length of time it will take for the waving solution to penetrate. The more porous the hair, the faster the penetration and the greater the chance for damage to the hair. (This is why those who color their hair should wait several weeks after the coloring before they have a perm.) As we age, even if our hair is not colored or treated in any way, the cuticle layer of the individual hairs no longer lies as flat as in youth, so it is more easily penetrated. The hair of older persons absorbs the perming solution faster than young hair does.

Thickness of your hair. The number of hairs on your head and the diameter of each of those hairs, as well as the way the hair is rolled on the forming rods, can make a difference in the tightness and bounce of a permanent. Thick hair and larger rods make for a looser permanent; thinner hair and smaller rods will result in a tighter permanent.

Here are some reliable perm products to use at home—after reading the directions very carefully:

- Extra Body Perm (L'Oréal)
- Kindness Curly Wave (Clairol)
- Premiere Perm (L'Oréal)
- Rave Extra Soft (Chesebrough-Ponds)

Permanent Mistakes

Most hair permanent mistakes are people errors. The manufacturers have tried hard to devise fail-safe, mistake-proof products that will give some success to even the most unskilled home hairdresser. But a few precautions are still necessary:

- Condition hair before perming.
- Roll equal amounts of hair on each rod.
- Work as quickly as possible and avoid any interruptions—seconds count.
- Apply the lotions as evenly as possible.
- Avoid an overprocessed front and an underprocessed back by planning which area should be treated first.
- Underprocessing is preferable to overprocessing—be conservative. If your hair is overprocessed, it will be frizzy, weak, dry, brittle, matted,

and, in the worst cases, gone. Underprocessing results in limp hair but is nowhere near as damaging.

- If you color your hair, make sure the label on the home perm indicates that it is safe for color-treated hair.

GMTG Sensitivity

Recently there has been an increasing problem with irritant and allergic reactions among both customers and hairdressers to an ingredient known as glyceryl monothioglycolate (GMTG). It is found in some of the acid neutralizers used in professional permanent kits. One way to identify GMTG is to look for kits containing three parts. The GMTG comes in a small tube and has to be mixed with the waving lotion. Operators, even those who wear protective gloves, have been known to have a reaction to this chemical. If the skin around the hairline is not protected with absorbent cotton and the neck with a towel, a burning irritation on the site of contact with the solution can occur almost immediately. Using a hair dryer can intensify this burn. An itchy reaction hours or days later anywhere on the face or neck is an allergic reaction, which you can alleviate with an over-the-counter antihistamine taken orally or topical steroid cream or lotion, such as Cortaid. You should also check with your dermatologist.

Permanent Care

Once you have given your hair a permanent, you will have to change your usual hair-care program to accommodate its new texture. Even the best of permanents are traumatic for the hair; the alkaline and acid solutions have stripped away its natural oils. The following is a program to help your hair recover:

- Use only a wide-toothed rubber or tortoise-shell comb; brush your hair less often and more gently.
- Select only acidic (low-pH) shampoos specially formulated for treated or damaged hair.
- Blot wet hair, don't rub it; avoid combing it until it is at least partially dry; never brush it when wet.
- Use a cream or protein conditioner to keep your hair shiny and smooth.
- Avoid hot blow dryers; air-dry your hair naturally, if possible.
- Use hot oil treatments if your hair is excessively dry; avoid drying situations such as direct sun, wind, and cold.

Both the strong perfumes used to mask the smell of the chemicals and the peroxides in the neutralizing solution can irritate the eyes. If any solution gets into your eyes, wash it away immediately with repeated applications of large quantities of lukewarm water. The neutralizers can be toxic if swallowed; caution should be taken to keep the products away from children. Use plastic or rubber gloves when applying the solutions to minimize contact with your skin.

The most important factor for the success of hair coloring or a permanent is the condition of your hair. You can't expect to get great results unless your hair is in good condition to start with. Good hair results from all the same things that good skin comes from: good genes, good nutrition, and sensible care. If your hair looks less than healthy, stop what you are doing to it and give it a vacation, not a permanent.

16

TWENTY PEARLY
SHIELDS—
HOW TO HAVE
HEALTHY NAILS

I love having my nails manicured. To me perfect nails are an essential part of good grooming. Within limits set by heredity and assuming reasonable care, your nails can be lovely adornments to your hands.

Nails and Cuticles—What Are They?

Nails, claws, hooves, horns, and hair are composed of the modified protein called keratin. Nails are semitranslucent horny plates. Like hair, nails are lifeless except at their roots. The roots are protected by the nail folds and cuticles.

You can trace your own nail growth by noticing any small mark or flaw in a nail and watching it move toward the tip. Care must be taken not to harm the base of a nail, since damage there can lead to a deformed nail.

Each nail is formed and starts its growth in an area under its cuticle called the matrix. The matrix is the only living part of the nail and its condition determines the appearance of the nail. The pale half moon at the base of the nail, called the lunula, is the visible portion of the matrix. Where the lunula ends, the nail bed begins. The pinkish color of the rest of the nail plate comes from the underlying network of small blood vessels seen through the almost translucent nail.

The hard nail plate, made of keratin, rests on the nail bed and is surrounded by three folds of skin, called nail folds—one at the base (proximal nail fold) covering the root, and two on the sides (lateral nail folds). Cuticles are U-shaped extensions of the proximal nail fold that are composed of dead horny cells. They keep objects and infectious organisms out of the nail bed.

Unlike hair that grows, rests, and then grows again, nails grow continuously through life and normally are not shed. Each nail on your hand grows at its own rate; the longer the finger, the faster the rate of nail growth. The nails of the two middle fingers grow faster than those of the thumb and little fingers. The nails on the dominant hand grow fastest, and toenails grow more slowly than fingernails. It takes five to six months for a fingernail to replace itself completely and up to a year or a year and a half for a damaged toenail to grow back. The average rate of fingernail growth is .5 to 1.2 millimeters per week.

The Five Commandments of Nail Care

Nails need the same sort of care you give your skin and hair. The cold weather and dry air that make your skin flake will also make nails brittle and prone to splitting. You can encourage healthy nails in the following ways:

1. Never use solvents or chemicals without protective gloves (this does your hands a favor, too). The best are cotton-lined rubber gloves.
2. Use a hand lotion, rubbing it into your nails as well as your hands as often as you can.
3. Don't dial; use a push-button phone or a phone dialer. Watch out for slamming doors, windows, and lids.
4. Avoid using your nails as tools to pry out staples, scrape up messes, tighten loose screws on your glasses, and perform similar mechanical tasks.
5. Be particularly careful of your nails after you have been outdoors in the cold; nails split most easily then. Always wear gloves in cold weather.

Nails grow faster in childhood, while you are in your twenties and thirties, during pregnancy, premenstrually, when the weather is hot, and after a minor injury. To speed the growth of your nails, you can tap your fingers, play the piano, type, or use a computer keyboard—these slight jarrings to the nails are enough to stimulate growth. Some illnesses, especially those associated with fever, and poor nutrition can slow nail growth. Nails also grow more slowly at night and in cold weather. Men's nails generally grow faster than women's.

Nail Problems

Brittleness

Do your nails break at the slightest provocation? Brittleness is often linked with age. Weak nails are a common postmenopausal problem, but they can also result from dryness and overexposure to such irritants as cleansers, soaps, detergents, solvents, nail polish removers, and insecticides. Other conditions that affect nails are:

• Iron deficiency anemia
• Impaired circulation
• Kidney problems
• Thyroid malfunction
• Stress (it affects everything)
• Osteoporosis

Brittleness is not due to dietary deficiencies; no evidence has been found to indicate that protein "nail builders" or gelatin, even in megadose capsules, affect nail strength. However, large doses (800–1,200 IU daily) of vitamin E taken orally for six months to one year have been effective in the treatment of yellowish nails and have also stimulated nail growth.

If your nails split easily, here is what you can do to make them more flexible:

• Soak your fingertips in warm water for about ten to fifteen minutes, then pat them dry.
• Rub each nail with olive or any mineral oil, petroleum jelly, or a moisturizer that contains phospholipids. I like New Formula Complex 15 Hand and Body Cream/Lotion (Baker/Cummins); it contains phospholipid-rich lecithin, a soybean product, and works wonders on nails. Creams with urea, such as Aquacare HP (Herbert), Nutraplus Lotion (Owen), and One and All (Innoxa), are also helpful.
• Cut nails while wet—after soaking in warm water for ten minutes—to minimize breakage.
• Wear nail polish or at least a base coat for protection.
• Use nail strengthening products as a base coat (Vital Nails' Develop 10 and Sally Hansen's Maximum Growth are two examples).

Nail Wrapping

Nail wrapping helps strengthen nails and prevents chipping as they grow out. For best results, glue sheer silk on the existing nail and then use a file to trim silk extending past the nail edge (cyanocrylate glue is usually used). If your nails are basically healthy, only one layer of silk is needed; weak or broken nails need added layers.

The reason nail wrapping works is that nails are made up of dead cells arranged in layers that can become separated and damaged if the nail is cracked. Nail wrapping holds these layers together, protecting the free edge and allowing it to grow forward without chipping. When the silk is finished with nail polish color and a top coat, the cloth reinforcement is totally undetectable.

Nails should be rewrapped at least once a month and will hold up best if a clear coat of polish is applied every couple of days. Nail color can be changed between wrappings.

Nail wrapping is not a good solution for anyone who washes her hands frequently or must immerse her hands in water for long periods. If you have a serious problem with splitting and peeling nails, consult your dermatologist.

Reaction to Medication

Nails are appendages of the skin, and the health of your nails and the health of your skin are related. It is possible that problems you may be having with your nails are the result of a medication you are taking. The antibiotic tetracycline and its relatives, widely used for acne and other skin infections, can produce a sun-sensitivity reaction that also causes the nails to loosen from their beds. A similar change is associated with the use of oral contraceptives. Anticancer agents and other medications can cause nail defects, too. If you are so affected, your doctor may be able to change your prescription and continue treating your condition while you save your nails. If you are using a medication known to produce phototoxic changes, wear a colored polish to protect nails from the sun.

Nail Biting

Nail biting is a common habit and not confined to children. Among its unpleasant effects are broken cuticles and warts around the fingernails. Nail biters are generally angry with their hands for looking so irritated, so it may help to set up a regular weekly grooming routine for manicures. It is an old truism that we love the parts we groom the most and groom and care for the features we like the most about ourselves. Being aware of your nails as objects of care may deter nibbling. Until your nails have regained a pleasing natural shape, avoid wearing bright nail colors. They will only draw attention to your nails' poor condition.

To help stop nail biting, you can apply plastic nails directly to the point where the nail has receded, even if the nail has been bitten down severely.

These artificial nails adhere with a soft plastic primer and can be filed to an attractive and comfortable length, then polished. A plastic nail can help to restore the sides of the damaged nail while protecting the new growth underneath. Since plastic nails don't seem as satisfying to bite as natural nails, they tend to discourage further biting. Applying clear nail polish may help deter biting, too, especially with children, who can't really wear plastic nails.

Like many other habits, you can cure nail biting by focusing on the situation or emotion that makes you bite. Do you do it when you're concentrating? When you're nervous? When you're bored or peeved? Getting rid of the triggers avoids many a problem and stops bad habits, too.

Hangnails and Damaged Cuticles

Hangnails are annoying, sometimes painful, small, hard triangle-shaped splits of skin at the sides of a fingernail. They are especially common among women who work with their hands in water or who bite their nails. Hangnails become infected if they are picked at. Cutting the cuticle with large or dull scissors, snagging it, or prodding it can also produce the problem.

As always, the best course is prevention: Keep your nails and the skin folds around them well moisturized. If a hangnail does develop, cut it off with narrow-bladed sharp scissors, being careful not to drag at it or poke at the live tissue to which it is attached. If you have a tendency to pick at hangnails when you're nervous, be sure that your clothes have pockets. Put one hand in each pocket and keep them there until the urge leaves.

Use caution with cuticle removing solutions, which are designed to deal with excess and raggedy cuticles. Since many of them contain sodium hydroxide, a caustic base that can destroy skin tissue, they can cause irritations if left on too long. When using a cuticle remover, follow the instructions on the package carefully. In any event, use such products sparingly, as cuticle has a vital protective function: to prevent harmful microorganisms from invading the nail matrix.

Aging

As noted, brittleness is often associated with nails as they age. Other age-related changes are:

- Thickening—including lack of uniformity, with alternating areas of thickening and thinning
- Vertical ridging, which is to nails what wrinkles are to skin.
- Absence of lunula—the disappearance of the white half moon on the bottom of the nail
- Opacity and brownish discoloration, although brown nails can also be caused by contact with walnuts, roasted coffee, or hydroquinone, the bleaching agent used for liver spots

Nail Cosmetics

Overuse of products intended to make the nails attractive—undercoats, polishes, and polish removers—can dry the nails to the splitting point. Used judiciously, however, polish actually protects your nails. Polishes that contain nylon fibers will add strength to your nails. However, most of us wear nail polish for aesthetic reasons.

Manicure

Learning how to give yourself a professional-quality manicure is like learning photo retouching: There's nothing inherently difficult about using any of the tools and procedures involved, but the work is hard to do well and it can't be rushed.

Here are some of the nail-care materials you will need for your manicure kit:

Emery board
Orangewood stick
Cuticle scissors
Cuticle nippers
Nail buffer
Oil for the cuticles (olive oil or
   baby oil)

Polish, enamel, or lacquer
Nail polish thinner or remover
Base coat
Top coat or sealer
Hand cream or a thick oily
   moisturizer

You will also need a small dish or saucer, absorbent cotton balls for removing polish, tissues, mending cloth, and paper. You may wish to add other tools that you find work well. Improvise—techniques, not professional tools, are more important.

Ten Steps to a Perfect Manicure

1. Remove old polish first with a cotton ball that is half saturated with remover. Follow up with a clean cotton ball barely moistened with remover to remove the last traces of polish. Rub the nail briskly so the remover will clean away the polish quickly and does not have time to penetrate too deeply. (Nails are made of many layers, and nail polish remover can penetrate them quickly, staining and drying the nail. Always work from the base of the nail to the tip, and try to avoid permitting color to lodge in the nail folds. It's best to use an oily nail polish remover to replace the oil you are stripping away. (To find an oily polish remover, look on the label—most manufacturers realize oil is a sales plus and announce it on the label.)

2. Rinse the nails and dry them carefully. Then, starting from your little finger and working toward the thumb of each hand, file your nails. Shape your nails so they complement the shape of your fingers and hands. File in one direction only, and hold the file so that the edge of the nail is beveled slightly. Finish off with a long sweeping stroke at a 45-degree angle. The beveling will strengthen the edges.

3. After filing your nails, soften your cuticles for two minutes by immersing your fingers in a bowl or saucer of warm soapy water to which a dash of baby oil or mineral oil has been added—or apply a heated moisturizer. Then rinse your fingers and dry completely. (To prevent dry cuticles, try Le Pont's Formula 405 nail treatment daily.)

4. As you dry your fingertips, *gently* push back the cuticles and adhering skin on each nail. If cuticles are handled too roughly, the matrix can be damaged, and white horizontal lines may develop on nails. If necessary, apply a cuticle remover around the cuticle of each finger, gently loosen the cuticle, and push it backward to reveal the pale half moon of the nail. Keep the cuticle moist while working to minimize chances of damaging it or the nail. (You may have heard that exposing the half moon makes the nail base vulnerable or that it is done for aesthetics only. Both are true. But pushing back the cuticle prevents it from growing excessively and becoming ragged.)

5. Clean under the free cuticle edge and around the side of the finger. Trim the cuticle if necessary, or use a hindo stone (a small, fine pumice shaped like a pencil) to carve it away. An uneven or ragged cuticle can encourage hangnails.

6. If you are not going to wear polish or plan to wear only clear polish, this is the time to use a whitener under the free edge of the nail. You can use zinc oxide, which is good for your nails, or a pencil that is simply a white pigment in a waxy substance (Alabastro from Borghese, for example).

7. If you are going to wear a colored polish, this is the time to apply the base coat that will prevent the color from your enamel penetrating and staining your nail. A base also fills in pits and smooths ridges. Apply the base coat with long strokes, starting with the little finger and moving toward the thumb.

8. Now add the polish. Work lightly and quickly, using sweeping strokes from the base to the edge of the nail. Work first on one side near the fold, then on the other near the opposite fold, saving the final stroke for the center of the nail. Or paint the tip first, then the rest of the nail.

9. Remove excess polish by dipping a cotton swab or cotton-coated orange stick into the remover and applying it carefully around the

cuticles and nail edges. To delay chipping remove a hairbreadth of polish around the tip of each nail with your fingertip or a bit of cotton. This is a professional trick that will help prolong the life of your manicure.

10. When the polish is slick to a light touch, apply a top or seal coat in the same manner. You can speed the hardening process by dipping your hands in ice-cold water. The nail enamel will harden instantly—but it won't last as long as an air-dried polish. Your manicure should last about a week. If your polish chips any sooner than that, spare your nails the dehydrating process of an extra manicure by repairing the flaw with a flick of the brush rather than starting over. To make your manicure last longer, apply a layer of top coat every other day. Applying a nail-strengthening product such as Develop 10 (Vital Nails) as both a base and top coat also makes a manicure last longer.

Allergic Reactions to Nail Products

Fortunately, allergic reactions to nail cosmetics are very rare. To avoid an allergic reaction it is best to choose a polish that is free of formaldehyde—but that is not always easy. Formaldehyde, a disinfectant, germicide, and fungicide best known for its use as an embalming fluid, is also used in nail polish formulas because it prevents nails from chipping, fragmenting, and peeling. Toluene sulfonamide/formaldehyde resin is the most common cause of skin reactions to nail products. Hypoallergenic polyester nail polishes such as Nail Polish (Almay) and Glossy Nails (Clinique) are free of this resin but do have a tendency to peel.

Tip: The chances of developing a formaldehyde reaction are reduced drastically once the nails have dried thoroughly, which is an argument in favor of using quick-drying products.

Nail polish can be responsible for allergic skin reactions not only on and around the nails themselves but also on the neck, eyelids (usually only one eyelid), face, and ears because many women tend to touch these areas before their nails are fully dry. The reactions on the facial areas resemble streaks of eczema; diagnosis can be difficult, as the cause seems so improbable. Possible allergens in nail polish include pigments, solvents, and plasticizers. Most polishes share certain common ingredients, but comparing labels will bring significant differences to light. (An allergic reaction can also occur on the leg, if a dab of polish is used to fix a pantyhose run.)

Buffing

Buffing is to nails what brushing is to hair. It stimulates them and encourages a good blood supply, making them pinkish in color. Buffing is exceptionally good for brittle nails; it also removes loose nail debris and smooths the nail plate. The appropriate frequency of buffing depends on the thickness of your nails: once a week for thick nails, and monthly for thinner ones. If your nails are strong and you are short on time to polish them, buffing gives a slight gloss and a groomed look.

Buffing powders are abrasive and should be used infrequently and cautiously. Keep an emery board with you at all times, however. Smoothing a tiny snag has saved many a nail—and also many pairs of pantyhose.

Artificial Nails

Among popular nail treatments are sculptured or porcelain nails, especially for those who like the look of very long nails. Nails are part of a total look; when you don't have great nails of your own, there are alternatives that can serve. (If your nails are very unhealthy, however, using artificial nails can be further damaging. See a dermatologist instead.)

Carefully read this entire section, including the information on problems with artificial nails, before you make any decisions about artificial nails.

- Never use artificial nails if your nails or the cuticles around them are infected.
- Never wear them for long periods of time. (Some manufacturers indicate time limits on their product's label.)
- Don't subject artificial nails to long periods of immersion in water.
- Be careful not to contaminate the adhesive holding the nails on with oil from a hand lotion or other substance.

Built-On (Sculptured) Nails

These are made by spreading a smooth-flowing, fast-drying mixture over a form or by actually reapplying your own broken nail to your finger. They are usually applied in the process of a manicure, just when you would normally apply a base coat of polish.

First the nail surface is roughened slightly with the fine side of an emery board. Then, using glue, the nail form is placed under the tip of the nail. A premixed plastic is painted on, slowly building the nail up until the desired length is reached. After filing away the excess, cleaning the sides of the nail of any mistakes, and generally neatening the nail with polish remover, the nail is allowed to dry. In about fifteen minutes it is ready to be polished.

Built-on nails can be removed with polish remover, but it requires time and the remover is very harsh on the real nail.

Press-On Nails

To apply press-on nails, follow this simple routine. Remove all old polish from your nails and manicure them up to the point at which you would apply new polish. Then roughen the nail surface slightly with the fine surface of an emery board and select the proper press-on nail size for each finger.

With sharp manicure scissors or a file, trim the artificial nail so that the cuticle end fits the shape of your natural nail. If the nail is too curved, flatten it by placing it under a book or heavy object for a few minutes or by reshaping it after heating in warm water.

Once the press-on nail is the right shape, apply a small amount of adhesive along the edges of your nail—avoid getting any adhesive on the center of the nail. Then apply adhesive to the inside edges of the press-on nail. Press the nail to your own, and hold it firmly for about a minute. Carefully wipe away any excess adhesive and complete the manicure by filing, shaping, and polishing the press-on nail.

To remove a press-on nail, use an oily polish remover. Avoid acetone removers, which can melt or deform the artificial nail's plastic. (Some nylon nails to not react to acetone; follow the directions on the manufacturer's box exactly.) After applying polish remover around the edges of the nail, gently lift the nail. Don't twist or pull it, as you can injure your own nail underneath. After press-on nails are removed, they can be stored for future use.

Problems with Artificial Nails

Artificial nails are usually built of an acrylic powder, a solvent, and instant glue. Applying them is a lengthy and not inexpensive process, but the same can be said of many beauty techniques.

The only really important problem with artificial nails is experienced by persons unlucky enough to develop allergic or irritant reactions, including tenderness, hemorrhaging under the nail, and the separation of the nail from the nail bed. In extreme cases the nail can fall off. In my practice, I've seen quite a few women whose nails have become deformed as a result of using artificial nails.

Both built-on nails themselves and the adhesives used to attach press-on plastic nails have the potential to produce allergic reactions. Although significant improvements have been made in adhesives, resins and glues made with cyanocrylates, commonly used for plastic nails, can be a problem. Since plastic or artificial nails are seldom used by persons whose natural nails are wonderful to start with, it is often hard to know whether the glues start trouble or simply add to a preexisting condition. Patch testing to determine sensitivity to the acrylic can help in diagnosis.

An allergic skin reaction never occurs at the first exposure to a substance, and the interval between the first exposure and the one that brings a reaction can vary from days to years.

Perhaps more common are fungal and bacterial infections that occur when the nail lifts from the bed. If a problem does occur, it may be several months—the time it takes for a new nail to grow out—before the nail looks normal again. Sometimes early injections of a steroid into the nail fold can prevent a permanent deformity. And monthly intralesional steroid injections can help if a deformity has already occurred.

What Your Nails Can Tell Your Doctor About Your Health

Doctors in ancient Arabia, not permitted to examine their female patients directly, sometimes based their diagnoses on nail analysis; the hands were the one part of their patient's anatomy they could inspect. Many of these doctors were amazingly accurate in detecting chronic health problems, and modern doctors can read the same signs.

- Spoon-shaped nails that bend upward at the base may be a sign of iron-deficiency anemia or coronary disease.
- Thickened nails with excessive ridging and splitting may indicate decreased blood circulation, perhaps due to hardening of the arteries.
- Overhanging nails and broad, thickened fingertips show lack of oxygenated blood.
- Clubbed fingers are among the signs of congenital heart disease.
- Separation of the nail plate from its underlying bed (onycholysis) may occur as the result of injury (including from excessive manicuring) or a long-standing fungal infection or psoriasis. Pregnancy and certain oral contraceptives may also cause this problem, as can diabetes, hyperthyroidism, hypothyroidism, and impaired circulation.
- Pitted nails are a common symptom of psoriasis and alopecia areata, a form of hair loss.
- Vertical ridges may indicate rheumatoid arthritis or Raynaud's disease, a condition in which the small arteries of the hands and feet go into spasms in response to the cold, cutting off circulation and, in severe cases, eventually causing small ulcers to develop on the fingertips.

Nail discolorations may also be special clues. Changes in nail color should not be ignored. (If your nails suddenly start to change color, chip, develop lines and ridges, or seem to loosen, consult a dermatologist.) Discolorations that follow the shape of the lunula usually have an internal cause; those that follow the shape of the cuticle tend to have an external cause.

- Blackish green—a bacterial infection
- Pale—anemia
- White transverse bands—chronic liver disease or arsenic poisoning; may also appear with each menstrual period
- Half and half (the tip is pink, the lower half is white)—kidney disease
- Dark streaks—a disorder of the adrenal glands
- Black splinters—an infection of the heart valves, scurvy, or chronic kidney disease
- White spots—calcium or zinc deficiency
- Yellow—vitamin D toxicity, diabetes, lung problems, thyroid disease, rheumatoid arthritis, or treatment with tetracycline

- Black—vitamin B$_{12}$ deficiency
- Blue-brown—caused by antimalarial drugs and often seen in those who have lived or been stationed in the tropics
- Red-brown—may come from using acne-fighting medication that contains resorcinol. (A pale red may simply mean color seepage from nail polish.)
- Red lunula—cardiac failure

Of course, not all discoloration is due to illness. Yellow nails can be the result of a slight stain left over from your nail polish, particularly if you use very dark polish or base coat. For dark yellow stains, buffing your nails will give them a glossy, natural finish while removing the surface yellow film. You can also bleach the nails slightly by rubbing them with a slice of lemon. However, if the yellow color persists, very likely it is being caused in some other way—possibly from smoking, bacterial or fungal infections of the nail, or exposure to certain dyes (particularly henna) or coal tar products.

Toenails

Ingrown Toenails

Ingrown toenails can hobble you. What happens is that the edge of the nail, instead of growing out normally into space, turns and penetrates the skin, causing an inflammation or "foreign body" reaction. This is often complicated by a bacterial infection.

Improper cutting of the toenails (straight across is the right way; never cut down the sides) and tight or ill-fitting shoes contribute to the problem. More men than women suffer from ingrown toenails, but pointed women's shoes, periodically reintroduced by fashion designers, often squeeze toes and nails to the extent that they cause ingrown nails. As the ingrown nail grows, the condition worsens.

It may be possible for you to treat an ingrown toenail yourself. Pack a piece of cotton or gauze between the nail and the flesh; change the dressing frequently until the soft tissue heals and the nail grows out. If an ingrown toenail does not respond to self-treatment, see your dermatologist without delay. Sometimes the nail has penetrated the flesh so deeply that surgical treatment is required. It may be necessary to cut away parts of both the nail and the adjoining flesh; in extreme cases the only cure is to have the nail removed. Sometimes silver nitrate, urea, salicylic acid, or potassium iodide in high concentrations are used instead of surgery.

Thickened Toenails

Most nail thickening occurs on the toes. It is quite rare on the fingers, although fingernails do thicken slightly with age and will also thicken if they are abused. If you constantly injure your nails, they attempt to protect themselves and thicken as a defense. (Examine the nails of a harpist or other musician who uses her nails and you will see thick nails.)

Heredity is the chief cause of thickened toenails, but you may be adding to the effect of your genes by failing to trim your nails properly and wearing shoes that constantly rub against the ends of the nails. If your nails are not treated, they can become hornlike and curve downward. Wearing shoes that are long enough with a toe box that is high enough and with an arch that fits correctly so your foot doesn't slide forward with each step is preventive therapy—and more comfortable besides.

Fungal Infections of the Toenails

Onychomycosis is a fungal infection of the nails, more often affecting the toenails than the fingernails. If you have a skin fungal infection such as athlete's foot, there is a 40 percent chance that you have this nail infection, too. Other predisposing factors include heredity, trauma to the nail, warmth and moisture, abnormal keratin of the nails (not unusual with age), diabetes, and chemotherapy. If you notice that your nails have become brittle, discolored (yellowish), thickened, crumbly, or separated from the nail bed—catching on clothing and looking so bad they embarrass you—you may have a fungal infection. See your dermatologist. Applying over-the-counter antifungal agents will not cure onychomycosis.

The condition is usually treated with an oral antifungal antibiotic (Griseofulvin) for the amount of time necessary for the nails to grow out—about six months for a fingernail infection, twelve to eighteen months for a toenail infection. If the condition is resistant to this antibiotic, the new prescription medication Nizoral (Janssen) can help. (Nizoral is also effective in the treatment of other types of fungal infections, including yeast.) Because onychomycosis tends to recur, topical antifungal creams should be used regularly as a preventive measure once the nails are cured.

In the early stages of fungal infection or as a preventive measure, you can apply the content of one vitamin E capsule to the nails daily.

Pedicures

A pedicure is to feet what a manicure is to hands. It can even make you walk better.

Pedicuring requires that you wash, moisturize, and examine your feet before caring for your nails. Check to see if you have developed calluses, corns, or ingrowing toenails. Athlete's foot and other conditions can be detected at this time.

You will need much the same equipment you used for your manicure and two basins of warm water, or use the tub if you are working in your bathroom. Lay out your tools so they are conveniently at hand when you begin.

Ten Steps to Happier Feet

1. Soak your feet in warm soapy water for about five minutes. You should have enough water to just about cover your ankles. Rinse and dry your feet carefully.
2. Use your pumice stone on hardened or callused skin on the soles or toes. Then apply moisturizing lotion and work it in around the nails and toes.
3. Remove any old polish from the nails of both feet. Avoid using too much polish remover and work from the base of the nail.
4. If trimming is necessary—generally every three to four weeks—trim the nails straight across with clippers or scissors. Leave them long enough to cover the ends of the toes.
5. File your toenails with your emery board. File straight across the tips, rounding them only slightly at the corners to conform with the shape of your toes. To avoid ingrown toenails, don't file the sides.
6. With a cotton-tipped orangewood stick, apply cuticle solvent to the cuticle and under the free edges of each toenail. Loosen the cuticles and gently push them down toward the base of the nail.
7. Rinse your feet, dry them carefully, and massage with hand cream. Massage your feet by sliding the thumbs and fingers along the foot and gently pulling on each toe. This softens the skin and improves circulation.
8. Remove all traces of cream and insert cotton balls, lamb's wool, or tissues between your toes preparatory to painting them.
9. Apply fresh nail polish, working from the cuticle up the nail. Allow as much time as possible for the nails to dry.
10. Apply witch hazel or a mild astringent to your feet with a cotton ball, and then sprinkle your feet with talcum powder to be sure your toes are completely dry before dressing or putting your feet into shoes.

You should be walking on easy street if you give yourself a weekly pedicure. It is especially important in winter, when you are most likely to forget. Attentive nail and foot care can keep your skin in good condition and your feet warmer because their circulation is better.

Nice Nails

Since your nails grow at the rate of about one-sixteenth of an inch each week, you can improve their looks quite easily. Of course, there is always one nail that chips or breaks. Treat that nail with just a bit more care than usual. Do your nail exercises daily (typing or word processing is exercise for nails). Most of all, watch your diet. Your nails, like your hair, respond to adequate nutrition (see the next chapter).

17

THE PROPER FEEDING
OF SKIN, HAIR,
AND NAILS

Your skin, hair, and nails grow from the inside out, and you have to feed them. They all depend on adequate nutrition.

What is adequate? The answer varies for different individuals, but some basics do not vary, and flouting them can affect your looks in just hours. Water, for example, makes a big difference in a short time. Nutrition is serious business if you care how you look.

The benefits of good nutrition begin to be ours as the foods we eat are assimilated in the digestive tract. Nutrients from food are dispersed in the bloodstream and in short order reach the smallest blood vessels of the body, the capillaries of the skin. A diet good for your skin will:

- Provide the nutrients you need to ensure the growth of new, healthy skin
- Minimize skin stress (stretch and strain) by keeping your body weight stable
- Provide adequate water for washing away wastes
- Repair damaged tissue by providing nutrients for healing. Slow healing, and a correspondingly greater chance of infection, may affect your total health. You need to keep your body's packaging as flawless as possible for total good health.

To keep your system running smoothly, which includes new skin cell production, you need just the right proportions of all nutrients.

Asking "What is a good food for my skin, hair, and nails?" is like asking what is the best color lipstick. A lovely pink can be great for one woman and disaster for another. No food by itself is good or bad. What makes a food good for you is the way it fits into your personal nutritional program and needs. In most cases, a diet to promote youthful, healthy skin is comprised of lots of fluid, fresh fruits, raw or minimally cooked vegetables, whole grains, and low-fat dairy products.

Can You Spot Your Dietary Deficiency?

A great many dietary deficiencies in this country are planned. They result from diets that have just one goal—to regulate body weight and girth—and fail to take objectives such as health and good skin into account. To my dismay, many of my women patients, concerned only about calorie counts, consume fewer than 1,500 calories a day. This can lead to serious nutritional deficiencies. I would guess half the women I know—or that you know—are on a weight reduction diet of some sort at this very moment.

Look through the list below and check problems that may apply to your own skin, nails, or hair. Are you eating yourself ugly? You may be able to turn the situation around with a trip to your local supermarket.

Problem	Possible Diet Connection
Dark-circled eyes	Not enough iron
Puffy eyes	Allergic reactions
Dry, rough skin	Lack of vitamins E or A
Easy bruisability	Deficiency of vitamins E, K, and/or C
Slow healing	Deficiency of vitamin K, vitamin C, or zinc
Thinning hair	Low protein or excess of vitamin A
Acne	Too much iodine or androgens
Pale skin with a yellowish tint	Deficiency of vitamin B_{12}
Hair loss and red scaliness of the face	Deficiency of zinc
Splitting nails	Deficiency of protein or calcium
Excessive oiliness of the face	Androgen-triggering foods or deficiency of vitamins B_2 or B_6
Premature graying	Deficiency of folic acid
Sagging	Deficiency of protein or vitamin C
Photosensitive dermatitis (pellagra)	Deficiency of niacin
Cracks on lip edges (mouth corners)	Deficiency of riboflavin (vitamin B_2) or vitamin B_6
Fatty tumors on eyelids	Too much cholesterol
Dilated capillaries	Very hot spicy food, excessive alcohol, or caffeine

How many problems can you check? If you can check even one it is time for a reexamination of your diet. Discuss your problem(s) with your physician or dermatologist to rule out other possible causes and to be sure whatever diet adjustments you make are appropriate. No one should make final decisions about nutritional needs based on a short checklist. This one has been presented only to suggest the range of connections that exist between diet and skin conditions.

To get a sense of the adequacy of your diet, you might want to start by keeping a diet diary. List your daily intake of foods against some of the information that follows.

What Are Women Made Of?

Skin is 70 percent water, 27 percent protein, 2 percent fat, 1 percent sugar; the rest is trace minerals such as calcium, an important factor for skin health. Like the other tissues of your body, skin is mostly water and protein, so ample quantities of both must be part of your diet.

The Primary Diet Components

Water

You can go without food for days or even weeks, but in some situations survival time without water can be twelve hours or less. Water is important in nearly all of life's chemistry, and the production, growth, and life of skin cells depend on it. Water is also essential for flushing away the body's chemical wastes. Water within the cells helps make your skin look smooth, firm, and tight.

We get some of the water we need from foods. Fruits and vegetables are on the average more than 80 percent water, meat is about half water, and even bread is moist. Women need about three ounces of water to process each ounce of food eaten. This translates into almost two quarts of water daily. Don't depend on food to supply your water needs; drink at least a quart and a half a day. You lose water even without perspiring—about one third of a quart per day is lost just by breathing.

When the weather is hot or you are very active, increase your water intake. The myth that you shouldn't drink water during vigorous exercise is a dangerous one. Drink one or two glasses of water before, during, and after exercise.

Not all beverages will satisfy your body's need for water. Caffeine and alcohol in particular are diuretics, increasing water loss and making you need extra water; a cup of coffee or a mixed drink is not a suitable thirst quencher.

Some people believe that drinking water before or during meals is harmful, but nothing could be further from the truth. Digestion begins in the mouth, where foods are broken into small particles and where enzymes in the saliva affect carbohydrates. Water speeds these processes. The digestion of protein also requires extra water intake.

Can you drink too much water? Not easily, because the brain has a water control center similar to the control that alerts the body to heat or cold. A dry mouth activates this mechanism. If you feel thirsty, drink. If you feel hungry, drink. Many women confuse the sensation of hunger and thirst, thus eating rather than drinking. Remember, water has no calories.

Protein

The proteins in human skin, hair, and nails are made from about twenty different amino acids. Most of us consume adequate amounts of complete proteins, foods that include all the needed amino acids, to satisfy our bodily requirements. Women generally need less protein than men; as little as two or three ounces daily are sufficient, although pregnant women and nursing mothers need more.

Most protein deficiencies can be traced to fad diets—fruit-only diets, liquid-only diets, or other bizarre food regimens. Vegetarians who disdain all animal food are also at risk.

Not all protein is the same. High quality protein, the kind with most of the essential amino acids, is found in lean meat, poultry, fish, dairy foods such as milk and cheese, and eggs. It is just what is needed for skin tissue growth and regeneration. However, excessive protein may lead to calcium depletion in the bones.

How to Find Your Personal Protein Needs

Most nutritionists agree that the average person needs about .42 grams of protein daily for each pound of body weight. If you weigh 100 pounds, you need about 42 grams of protein a day; if you weigh 200 pounds, you need about 84 grams; and if your weight is in between, you can easily estimate your personal protein need.

A small daily serving of protein will be adequate for most women. You can get too much of any good thing. When you eat a very high-protein diet, you may also be ingesting too much fat or cholesterol, especially if you eat beef, some cuts of pork, lamb, shellfish, or deli meats.

Carbohydrates

The chief source of human fuel is carbohydrates, or sugars and starches. The body burns carbohydrates preferentially to produce the energy needed for movement and work. However, if a diet supplies insufficient carbohydrates to meet energy needs, the body may begin to metabolize (burn up) its own proteins, with disastrous consequences for the skin, nails, and hair. The connection between carbohydrate intake and the health of your skin is indirect but important; you need to eat carbohydrates to limit the burning of protein for energy.

Fat

Fat is a necessary part of the body's fuel. Because of undeserved bad press, many women are too wary of this essential nutrient. Besides serving as an important source of energy to protect the body's proteins, fats have many additional functions in your body. Layers of fat just under the skin provide insulation and, incidentally, account for most of the lovely curves we regard as essential to feminine beauty. Fats are also a medium for supplying necessary fat-soluble vitamins to the body and serve as part of cell structure. When digested, fats break down into several types of fatty acids vital to cell growth and skin health.

How Much Fat Before You Get Fat?

Estimates vary about how much fat most American women eat. Some researchers believe that the average diet of American women is now more than 50 percent fat. A high-fat diet may lead to a variety of problems, including breast and colon cancers. Most nutritionists suggest that fat be limited to no more than about a third of the calories in your total daily intake. The aim is not to eliminate fat from the diet, but to limit it.

Polyunsaturated fats, the most essential sources of fatty acids, are found in grains, nuts, some vegetables, sunflower seeds, and corn and safflower oil. If your diet is too low in these important fats, your skin will be dry and scaling. (An oily diet does not give you oily skin. The oil produced by your skin's oil glands reflects hormone levels, not fat in your bloodstream.)

Changes in the amount of fatty acid intake can affect the course of such common disorders as psoriasis. For example, low arachidonic acid diets (avoiding eggs, red meat, and some oils) and high eicosapentanoic acid diets (coldwater fish such as cod, haddock, and mackerel and fish oil) improve psoriasis.

Fiber

How food is used and how waste is processed are also important for your total health and your skin's look of vibrance and beauty.

In the past dozen years there has been a revolution in breakfast cereals: Almost all the popular brands now stress fiber. All fibers are not the same. Some that make up the walls of plants are insoluble in water and cannot be digested by bacteria in the digestive system. Most of these insoluble fibers can absorb many times their own weight in water and tend to speed movement of food through the body. They are supplied in most diets by wheat bran found in whole grain cereals. Pectins, which slow the movement of food passing through the system, are another type of fiber. Most pectins are supplied by the food additives, thickeners, and stabilizers found in almost all processed food.

Aim for approximately 40 grams of dietary fiber a day. If you need to, add fiber to your diet slowly and drink plenty of fluids along with eating raw or slightly cooked vegetables. Because fiber absorbs a great deal of water internally, when you eat more fiber you must remember to drink more water, too.

Fiber is not a cure-all. Even with additional fiber, a diet low in proteins, vitamins, and minerals will still be a poor diet.

Minerals and Vitamins

If fats, carbohydrates, and proteins were all the nutrients we needed, we could cook up a stew of steak, sugar, and oil and stay healthy forever. Life is more complicated than that. Besides protein and fuel for energy, we need a range of vitamins and minerals. While the exact functions of many of these special substances are not completely understood, their presence or absence can make all the difference in how you look and feel.

The following lists show some of the ways that minerals and vitamins affect the body and indicate some of their known dietary sources. These listings provide general health details as well as skin-care information. By looking through them you can spot some of the causes of problems that you may have checked on the problem-identification list given on page 199.

Minerals

Calcium

Calcium is the most abundant mineral in the body; 98 percent of it is found in the bones and teeth. Besides giving firmness and rigidity to bones and teeth, it activates enzymes and is vital to the clotting of blood and to muscle and nerve functioning—including the contractions of the heart—and can correct fingernail splitting seen in osteoporosis. The average person should consume just under one gram a day, but thin, active women should consume much more to avoid osteoporosis. Pregnant women, nursing mothers, smokers, alcohol and caffeine drinkers, and those under stress also need more.

Sources: dairy products, kale, broccoli, dark greens, almonds, Brazil nuts, oysters, canned salmon and sardines, mineral water, kidney beans, cabbage. If you take calcium supplements, make sure they are calcium carbonate (500 milligrams twice a day is the average recommended dosage).

Phosphorus

Essential for the metabolism of fats and carbohydrates, phosphorus also works with calcium in connection with the muscles, nerves, bones, and teeth and is essential to brain function. An increase in calcium in your diet requires a corresponding increase in phosphorus.

Sources: dried beans, peas, liver, meats, peanuts, brown rice, eggs, whole grains and cereals, many soft drinks.

Iron

Vital to the formation of hemoglobin, which carries oxygen from the lungs to the tissues of the body, iron is also essential for a healthy complexion, hair, and nails. The body actually contains less than 4.5 grams of iron, compared with about 125 grams of potassium and 25 grams of magnesium, but there is a constant need for this mineral—especially in pregnant and menstruating women—and storage is limited. Eat foods containing iron every day. A deficiency can cause fatigue, pale skin, generalized itching, canker sores, hair loss, and spooned (concave), soft or brittle fingernails.

Sources: organ meats, greens, spinach, wheat germ, bran, raisins, egg yolks, potatoes, poultry, shellfish, beans, tomato juice, nuts, dried apricots and prunes, pasta, fortified white bread, cereals.

Sodium

Sodium is found in the blood, serum and lymph fluids, and tissues of the body. It is a balancer between calcium and potassium and other minerals and prevents excessive loss of moisture from tissues. High-sodium diets can lead to water retention, hypertension, and stroke. Some sodium salts are excreted in the urine, but most are lost through sweating and should be replaced quickly or nausea, diarrhea, and cramps can result. Avoid excess salt.

Sources: salt, bananas, crackers, cheese, fish, pickles, buttermilk, bacon, canned corn, beets, crab, the flavoring MSG (monosodium glutamate).

Potassium

This mineral is important to the functioning of the nervous system in particular and in many other ways as well. A lack of potassium can make you feel weak and dizzy.

Sources: bananas, dried beans, meat, prunes, raisins, spinach, avocados, carrots, pears, oranges, grapefruits, nuts, melons, potatoes, tomatoes, yogurt, brussels sprouts.

Magnesium

Magnesium is important for the function of nerves and muscles and as an aid to the absorption of other minerals.

Sources: milk, greens, cabbage, liver, apples, nuts, seafood, corn, fish.

Manganese

Manganese is essential in the body's use of oxygen and the growth of bones and tendons. It is needed for proper functioning of the liver, kidney, and pancreas. A deficiency can cause problems with sexual functioning, especially in the development of sexuality; an excess can be toxic.

Sources: beef, beans, blueberries, dates, rice, nuts, wheat germ, tea, pears, coffee

Sulfur

Essential for healthy skin, hair, and nails, sulfur is required for the synthesis of body proteins. Sulfur bonds are responsible for naturally wavy hair.

Sources: lean meats, fish, egg yolks, potatoes, dried beans, cabbage, cauliflower, brussels sprouts, wheat germ, clams, onion, garlic, peanuts.

Chloride

Essential to normal gastric secretion and the processing of foods, chloride is also important in muscle action and balances acids and alkali levels in the blood.

Sources: salt, cottage cheese, milk, pasta, eggwhite, fish, ripe olives, pickled and smoked meats.

Copper

Copper functions with iron to produce hemoglobin. It also plays an important role in collagen formation. Insufficient amounts can cause anemia and changes in the color and structure of hair. Too much can change the color of the mucosa inside the mouth. An overdose is possible from the long-term use of copper pots for cooking.

Sources: beans, lobster, shrimp, oysters, green vegetables, nuts, liver, kidney, margarine, raisins, chocolate, meat, corn oil.

Iodine

Although important for healthy skin and thyroid functioning, too much iodine can bring on acne.

Sources: seafood, vegetables grown in iodine-rich soil (found in the southeastern United States), whole wheat, peanuts, wheat germ, kelp, saltwater fish, sea salt, some hamburgers and French fries cooked in iodine-sterilized utensils.

Fluoride

Fluoride modifies calcium and phosphorus metabolism and is important to healthy bones and teeth. In excess, it can cause mottling of teeth.

Sources: milk, cabbage, fluoridated water, whole wheat, seafood, tea, dry legumes. Fluoride is naturally present in the water in some areas of the United States.

Zinc

Zinc is important in skin metabolism, protein synthesis, and tissue repair. Deficiency can cause hair loss, scaling of hands and feet, dermatitis, slow healing, white streaks on nails. Zinc sulfate taken orally can promote skin healing. Too much zinc may cause drowsiness, muscle pain, and impaired immune response.

Sources: meat, poultry, seafood, eggs, milk, popcorn, whole corn, hard cheese, nuts, peas, beans, wheat germ, iron-rich foods.

Other Minerals

Various other mineral elements are also essential for good health, including selenium, an anticarcinogen and antioxidant (taken orally, it may also improve acne), and vanadium, which helps promote growth.

However, some trace minerals that find their way into food or water can be dangerous. Mercury residues can cause severe neurological damage and should be avoided whether in foods or as ingredients in creams or cosmetics. Cadmium, which is present without a counterbalance in processed white wheat flour, has been implicated in the development of heart attacks.

Vitamins

Vitamins are regulators of body functions. Since few of them can be manufactured by the body, we must acquire them by eating foods that contain them. Only very tiny quantities of each are required—a day's supply of them all would fill less than one-eighth of a teaspoon. The frantic pursuit by many people for the right vitamins in the right amounts has given rise to a huge industry and an endless din of claims and counterclaims. In this case, where there's smoke, there's fire: Vitamins are extremely important to good health.

Vitamin A

Vitamin A is fat soluble. It is destroyed by high temperature and exposure to the air, a consideration relevant to the way you cook. Store any source of vitamin A in a cool, dark place. Vitamin A is important for healthy skin, hair, and mucous membranes and is essential for visual function; it is also involved in the metabolism of fat. New evidence indicates that it has anticarcinogenic and antioxidant properties. A deficiency of vitamin A results in rough, scaly, wrinkled skin, goosebump-like accentuations of the hair follicles, dry and brittle hair, dry eyes, and a tendency to night blindness. Too much may cause dry, itchy skin, dry lips, hair loss, or yellowish skin tint. An excess can be toxic, even lethal. (The livers of certain large fish and of fish-eating polar bears contain such large concentrations of vitamin A that those livers are poisonous.)

Sources: Fish-liver oils are highly concentrated sources; yellow and orange vegetables have carotene, which the body converts into vitamin A. It is also found in liver, milk, butter, margarine, and apricots. 100,000 I.U. of vitamin A taken daily for a few weeks, under a physician's direction, will help oily skin and large pores.

Vitamin B₁ (Thiamine)

This is a water soluble vitamin, impaired by high temperatures. It helps your body metabolize carbohydrates. Persons who eat significant amounts of sugar, drink lots of alcohol, and burn up large amounts of energy in exercise and women using oral contraceptives may need thiamine supplements. Thiamine also helps the nervous system. Deficiencies are not specific; loss of appetite and indigestion is sometimes an indication. In high doses it interferes with absorption of other B vitamins.

Sources: pork, oysters, yeast, whole grains, oatmeal, lima beans, brewer's yeast.

Vitamin B₂ (Riboflavin)

Also water soluble and impaired by high temperatures, riboflavin helps your body use carbohydrates and proteins. It is very important for healthy skin and hair. Deficiencies can lead to cracked and chapped lips, excessive oiliness of the face, scaliness around the nose and mouth, cracks at the corners of the mouth, and in severe cases, loss of hair, burning tongue, and genital lesions. If you exercise a lot or take oral contraceptives, you need extra B_2.

Sources: mushrooms, milk, whole grains, liver, lean meat, leafy vegetables, yogurt.

Vitamin B₃ (Niacin)

Another water soluble vitamin impaired by high temperatures, niacin is present in all tissues and important chemically in the use of oxygen. It provides nutrients to hair cuticle. Deficiency may lead to pellagra, a disorder characterized by dermatitis (rashes on the face and tops of the hands or other parts of the body exposed to the sun), diarrhea, and dementia (mental deterioration). Half an hour after taking as little as 50 milligrams a flush may appear on the face. Large doses can cause flushing of the face and upper body and should be avoided by women with acne rosacea or thin, sensitive skin; too much can also cause brown pigmentation.

Sources: eggs, meat, liver, cereals, poultry, peanuts.

Vitamin B₆ (Pyridoxine)

Pyridoxine helps in the formation of red blood cells and proteins, the use of fats, and keratin production. Deficiencies may lead to anemia, cracks at the corners of the mouth, excessive oiliness of the face, susceptibility to infection, seborrhea-like lesions, scaling, and change in color of hands and feet. A mild deficiency caused by oral contraceptives or stress can bring on a mild depression. The more protein you eat, the more pyridoxine you need. Your body adjusts to high doses so that when they are lowered to normal levels, deficiency symptoms can manifest themselves.

Sources: lean meats, poultry, green vegetables, green beans, avocados, bananas, whole grains, potatoes.

Vitamin B₁₂

This vitamin helps to synthesize genetic material and form red blood cells; it is vital for the functioning of the nervous system. Pale lemon yellow skin, numbness, tingling in the fingers and toes, loss of balance, weakness, and anemia can signal deficiencies, as can oral paresthesias (abnormal sensations). Strict vegetarians who eat no animal foods at all are vulnerable to deficiency, as are women using oral contraceptives.

Sources: liver, kidney, eggs, oysters, other foods of animal origin.

Pantothenic Acid (a B Group Vitamin)

Pantothenic acid assists tissue metabolism and is involved in the functions of the nervous system. Stunted growth, dermatitis, gray hair, personality changes, and numbness in the fingers and toes have been traced to deficiencies. Too much can cause water retention and diarrhea.

Sources: liver, kidney, whole grains, nuts, eggs, and dark green vegetables.

Para-aminobenzoic Acid (PABA)

PABA protects skin from damaging ultraviolet light rays. (It is the main ingredient in most sunscreens.) In animal studies the combination of PABA and folic acid has successfully reversed graying of hair.

Sources: liver, kidneys, brewer's yeast, wheat germ, yogurt.

Biotin

This B complex vitamin helps form the fatty acids and metabolize proteins, fats, and carbohydrates. It stimulates hair growth. Persons with biotin deficiencies are listless and complain of weak muscles and poor coordination as well as scaly scalp and hair loss, pale skin, and cracked, red tongue. Consuming large amounts of raw egg white can destroy biotin (which is present in the egg yolk); cooked egg whites do not have this effect.

Sources: egg yolks, liver, kidney, green beans, sardines, brewer's yeast, whole grains.

Folic Acid

A B complex vitamin, folic acid acts with vitamin B_{12} in synthesizing genetic material, aids in the formation of red blood cells, and offsets pigmentary changes. It is very important for women who have a tendency to iron deficiency anemia. Women using oral contraceptives, pregnant women, nursing mothers, and those who use aspirin and alcohol may need extra folic acid. Folic acid deficiency can cause dull hair, premature graying of hair, and brownish skin pigmentation. Too much can cause sleep disturbances and irritability.

Sources: dark, leafy vegetables, broccoli, wheat germ, dried beans, raw fruits, meat, liver.

Vitamin C (Ascorbic Acid)

Vitamin C aids in the formation of collagen and helps maintain strong body tissue, cartilage, teeth, and bones. It increases absorption of iron and folic acid, promotes healing, repairs injured hair follicles, and is considered an anticarcinogen. Scurvy, slow-healing wounds, morning puffiness of the eyes, swelling of the legs, bruises, bleeding gums, and rough, discolored, dry skin with prominent follicles are symptoms of deficiency. Smokers, older people, women taking birth control pills, and aspirin and tetracycline users need extra vitamin C. Injury, stress, and surgery also increase the need for vitamin C.

Sources: citrus fruits, tomatoes, melons, green peppers, dark green vegetables, strawberries.

Vitamin D

Vitamin D is fat soluble but withstands heat well. It is made in the skin by sunlight—fifteen minutes outdoors a day meets the body's requirement for vitamin D, although it is also found in many foods. Required for the proper use of calcium and phosphorus in forming and maintaining teeth and bones, vitamin D is also considered an antioxidant and anticarcinogen and may play a role in regulating skin pigmentation. Muscle spasms, twitching, soft, fragile bones, and a deformed skeleton can result from insufficient amounts. Megadoses can result in the demineralization of the bones, calcium deposits in the kidneys, and excess calcium throughout the body (the body can't utilize vitamin D without calcium). Vitamin D has recently been found to have some sunscreening properties.

Sources: milk, cod liver oil, tuna, salmon, egg yolks, liver, sardines, herring.

Vitamin E

Vitamin E is also fat soluble and withstands heat. It prevents abnormal breakdowns in body tissues, helps form red blood cells, and is an antioxidant. Vitamin E increases vitamin A absorption and its effect. High doses of vitamin E have a photoprotective effect. Vitamin E has some anti-inflammatory properties. Used topically it acts as a moisturizer, may prevent scarring, and can suppress sun-induced redness. A deficiency is seldom seen in women except after prolonged avoidance of all fats as part of excessive dieting. However, estrogen-dominant birth control pills and laxatives interfere with its absorption. Insufficient vitamin E may lead to dry, rough skin and easy bruising. Megadoses make nails grow faster, but too much can result in chapped lips, hives, fatigue, and depression.

Sources: vegetable oils, whole grains, dried beans, liver, leafy green vegetables, wheat germ, corn.

Vitamin K

Taking antibiotics may have undesirable side effects, one being to kill the population of normal intestinal flora along with the targeted pathogens. At such times vitamin K, normally produced in sufficient amounts by the flora within the body, becomes a concern and supplements must be taken. Vitamin K is vital to the process of normal blood clotting (its name comes from the German word *Koagulation*) and is essential for skin healing. That is why supplements are given when a surgical procedure is imminent. Vitamin K deficiency manifests in easy bruisability.

Sources: most foods, but especially spinach and other leafy vegetables, tomatoes, eggs, liver.

Dieting

The average woman's body weight is about 25 percent fat; the average man's about 16 percent fat. If your fat weight is a higher percentage than this of your total body weight, you should restrict your food intake—in other words, go on a diet. Unfortunately, it is not easy to determine the ratio of fat to total body weight.

Overweight women are often depressed about being fat and tend to neglect the care of their skin, hair, and nails, among other things. Heavy women also suffer specific skin problems. They can be affected by intertrigo, an irritation of skin folds in the groin, at the armpits, and beneath the breasts—in any area that is constantly moist and warm (see chapter 12). Cellulite, a condition many claim has been invented by beauty entrepreneurs, is nevertheless evident on the thighs of many overweight women.

I believe you should deal with excess weight by both dieting and exercising. A pound of body fat contains about 3,500 calories. To lose a pound of weight, a person must use up 3,500 calories more than she takes in. When less food is eaten, the intake of calories goes down, but so does the intake of vitamins, minerals, and water. A dieter needs to drink more water than usual and, in some situations, to take vitamin and mineral supplements. You should consult your own physician when trying to lose weight or use supplements, because self-prescribed megadoses of nutrients can touch off eruptions of acne and other skin problems.

Skin, Hair, and Nail Cuisine

Lists of foods and special diets help to guide you to the right nutrition for your skin needs. The problem is, who can always abide by the lists? Many women eat out at least once every day. Most restaurant menus provide only a very limited number of foods that are suitable for skin-, hair-, and nail-loving diets. Here are a few general suggestions for dealing with many menus.

Fast-food restaurants. Avoid fried foods. The problems associated with them are more the result of utensils cleaned with iodine-related disinfectants than with the fat they contain, but the fat can be a problem, too. Iodine cleansers leave enough residue to stimulate oil glands and cause an acne flare-up. Broiled burgers are better than fried.

Chinese food. The Chinese system of cuisine uses five basic cooking methods: steaming, broiling, stir-frying, roasting, and simmering. Steaming is the best method for health and skin (no oil is added). Food is placed on a bamboo rack over a wok of boiling water; steamed vegetables, fish, and chicken are prepared in this way. Chinese cooks use several sauces. Avoid soy sauce if possible, as it is highly salty. Szechuan and Hunan dishes are spicier and hotter than Mandarin or Cantonese dishes and may cause skin flushing.

East Indian food. Ghee, a clarified liquid butter, is eaten with many dishes; avoid it. Also pass on spicy curried dishes. Tandoori chicken (broiled and dry) is a good choice.

French food. The organ meats—sweetbreads, brain, kidneys—are not for you if you have any tendency to blemishes. Light white wine sauces rather than cream sauces will spare you calories. Country dishes such as cassoulet, made with beans and pork, are rich in iron but also potential troublemakers for those with a tendency to acne rosacea. Also avoid pâté de campagne, made with pork and liver and highly seasoned and fatted. The cheeses of France are among the world's most inviting, but try to avoid them, as well as France's famous red wines (they dilate the capillaries of the face), especially if you are prone to rosacea. Select fresh fruit, white wine, and a light fresh bread rather than a buttery croissant.

Italian food. Pasta, rice, and fresh greens are fine, but cheese sauces and shellfish are troublemakers for the acne-prone. Veal is less fatty than beef and an excellent substitute for chicken. The tomato-thickened sauces of southern Italy can be included in most diets. Eat plain pizza to avoid the preserved meats and spices heaped on some varieties, and wait until the pizza cools slightly. Hot food stimulates oil glands and also flushes your face.

Russian food. Steaming borscht in the winter or chilled borscht in the summer, made with either a beef or chicken stock, will cause few problems, but blinis made with a yeast-heavy dough and covered with caviar may stimulate acne.

Mexican food. High seasoning and the lack of green vegetables are potential troublemakers for any complexion. Drinking water is a must during or after any Tex-Mex barbecue. (The high-protein meat and beans and the spicy seasoning need to be diluted so they are easier to digest.) Although smoked foods are quite popular, the crusty charcoal on the outside of the meats has been linked with serious stomach problems.

Special Diets

Most people need a well-balanced normal diet, but some of us suffer skin reactions to certain otherwise nutritious and healthful foods. Here is a list of foods which, though either harmless or positively nutritious for most people, may pose problems for others. Following that is a list of foods that help women maintain health and promote beauty. I often give my patients simple lists of foods that they should avoid or select. It gives them a handy reference when they are eating in a restaurant, shopping for food, or planning a menu at home. Note that some foods are included in both lists— you have to weigh their benefit to you against a possible disadvantage.

Foods That Sometimes Cause Problems

Acne triggers—foods that can add unwanted androgens or iodine to your diet if you are prone to acne

Shellfish
Peanut butter
Wheat germ
Gluten bread
Organ meats (liver, kidneys, sweetbreads)
Steroid-fed chickens

Peanuts
Whole-wheat flour
Iodized salt
Eggs in large quantities
Cheese (except skim milk cottage cheese)

Rosacea triggers—foods that can bring a flush to your face if you are sensitive

Beer, red wine, sherry
Spicy foods and beverages
Avocados, bananas, pineapples
Sharp aged cheeses
Caffeinated drinks

Relish
Raw onion
Mustard
Ketchup
Monosodium glutamate (MSG)
Tomatoes

Processed meats
Chocolate
Citrus fruits
Pickled herring
Nuts

Hot foods and beverages can also bring a flush to your face. Allow them to cool slightly before eating.

Edema triggers—foods that can encourage water retention

Salted pork
Smoked foods
Goose
Soups (bouillon cubes)
Baked beans

Fried foods
Duck
Shellfish
Gravies
Canned vegetables

Bacon
Herring
Soy sauce
Caviar
Pickles

| Quiche | Salted nuts | Dried beef |
| Olives | Processed cheeses | Canned tuna |

Allergy triggers—foods often known to inspire an allergic reaction, including occasional hives or asthma

Fried foods	Chocolate	Soy
Milk	Nuts	Plant foods
Shellfish	Peanuts	Fowl
Fish	Tomatoes	Pink peppercorns
Strawberries	Sauces	(related to poison ivy)
Eggs	Veal	

Photosensitizing foods—contact with lips or skin makes them more sensitive to the sun's rays

Limes (especially juice)	Parsnip	Dill
Oranges	Parsley	Mustard
Figs	Lettuce	Onion
Cinnamon	Artichokes	Garlic
Cucumber	Fennel	Horseradish
Corn	Carrots	Chives
Asparagus	Celery	Okra

Odor makers—foods that tend to stimulate odor in perspiration

Beer and other alcoholic beverages	Vinegar
Garlic and onions	Sharp cheeses
Hot spices	Organ meats
Eggs	Mustard

Foods That Promote Health

Bone food

Loss of bone mineral content, osteoporosis, is a common problem of postmenopausal women. Exercise, calcium in the diet, and vitamin D supplements are necessary. Bone thinning leads to smaller bone mass and saggy skin.

Canned salmon	Oranges	Whole milk
Sardines (especially the bones)	Skim milk	Oysters
	Cheese	Broccoli
Herring	Spinach	Ice cream
Yogurt	Kale	Almonds
Collard greens		

Anemia fighters—foods rich in iron
(Note that some iron-rich foods are high in cholesterol.)

Pork	Liver	Chili beans
Lamb	Carrots	Lentils
Shellfish	Apricots	Kidneys
Spinach	Eggs	Squash
Dark chicken and	Split peas	Raisins
turkey meat	Lean beef	

Hair and nail growers—protein-rich foods with varying fat content

Skim milk	Cottage cheese	Fish, especially
Salmon	Yogurt	haddock
Liver	Dried beans	Poultry
Wheat germ	Nuts	Eggs
Lean beef	Peanut butter	Mushrooms

Hives and Other Food Allergies

Hives (urticaria) are itchy red welts that occur almost anywhere on the skin. They appear without warning and often subside just as quickly. Most hives are caused by food allergies, although anxiety can also be a cause. Some nice detective work is required to find the source. The most common culprits are:

Milk	Cheese	Beef
Chocolate	Strawberries	Eggs
Wheat	Oranges	Soy
Nuts	Seafood	

Any foods that contain even a small amount of these reaction-producing ingredients can cause hives in some people. A piece of cake that is made with eggs can cause an egg reaction. The artificial sweetener aspartame, known as NutraSweet, has been incriminated as an occasional cause of urticaria. Most food allergy reactions occur immediately or within a few hours and can be accompanied by vomiting, abdominal pain, diarrhea, or asthma.

The itchy welts almost always subside spontaneously, so no treatment at all may be the best treatment in some cases. If you are uncomfortable, over-the-counter antihistamines such as Chlor-Trimeton (Schering) or Benadryl (Parke-Davis) usually bring relief. Since anxiety is often a contributing cofactor, relaxing your life-style a little can also help.

Allergies have a variety of interesting interrelationships. If you are allergic to certain foods you might also be allergic to others: If you are allergic to peanuts, then you may be allergic to soybeans; to cola nuts (used as a flavoring in soft drinks), then also to chocolate; to beef, then also to milk. The symptoms of food allergy are quite specific: Eggs usually produce hives; citrus fruits, eczema; and chocolate, headaches. A wholly hypoallergenic diet would include little more than water, lamb, rice, sugar, beans, and apples.

Sulfite allergies are especially common among asthma sufferers. The manifestations are itching, hives, even asthma attacks. Sulfites preserve food freshness and until recently were used in some restaurants (on salads and salad bars, for example), in packaged foods (check the labels), and in some medications such as bronchodilators. Sulfites are now widely prohibited for food preservation purposes.

18

SMOOTH FLYING AND

PRETTY LANDINGS

I love to travel; for me nothing is more exciting. New places, new faces, even the change in the color of the sky and trees is wonderful and refreshing. Last year I went to Switzerland for just a few days and I found the trip refreshing and restful, probably because I invested some time in preflight and in-flight self-care.

Businesswomen attend conventions, make sales calls, close million-dollar deals, and attend rounds of corporate meetings thousands of miles from home. Many of my patients travel several times a year; some travel several times a month. Frequent travelers usually develop a routine that lets them have smooth takeoffs and emerge from the plane looking great.

Preflight Preparations

Your preparations for a long flight should start well before you leave for the airport. Start preparing yourself against fatigue a month ahead of time by making sure that you have adequate vitamin C (60 milligrams a day—equal to one serving of citrus fruits) and calcium (1,500 milligrams a day—try to include a glass of whole, skim, or low-fat milk and a slice of hard cheese or heaping tablespoon of cottage cheese in that daily requirement).

Vitamin C counters the effects of ozone toxicity; calcium increases oxygen absorption. High-flying planes are low in oxygen, and you need to be able to use all the oxygen that is available.

If your trip will carry you through several time zones, consult chapter 12 of *Managing Your Mind and Mood Through Food* by Judith Wurtman (Rawson Associates, 1986). Entitled "Travelers' Advisory: Anti–Jet Lag Tactics," it tells exactly what to eat before departure, during flight, and afterward, when traveling east to west, west to east, or through an unusual number of time zones, which can be very depleting and thus destructive to your looks (not to say your ability to enjoy yourself or to work upon arrival).

Packing Cosmetics and Toiletries

No matter where you are heading or what clothing you are taking, there are some basics that you will need. You will certainly need cosmetics and some of your own favorite skin-care equipment. (I have wasted precious time in hotel pharmacies trying to find a substitute for a forgotten soap or shampoo.)

Here is how to pack up your cosmetics and toiletries.

Estimate your needs. To learn how much shampoo or any other item you will need to take, use your travel containers at home for a few weeks and see how much they hold. You will get used to them and discover any problems with the products.

Use glass containers. Don't use plastic containers from the drugstore, as cheap plastics may react with the chemicals in your cosmetics, especially in the case of astringents and fresheners. Finding enough small-sized glass jars is a never-ending problem unless your town has a chemical supply store that stocks them. Samples given out when cosmetic companies have specials usually are ideal.

Leave space on top. Do not fill your containers to the top; leave space for expansion and contraction as the pressure changes. When packing, use a large cosmetic bag with a waterproof lining as protection against leakage and insulation against breakage.

Keep your cosmetics nearby. Try to keep your regular daily makeup articles in a makeup kit that will fit in your hand luggage for touch-ups. (I have found that some of the least expensive kits work the best and can be replaced easily when that inevitable stain or spill occurs. I also think that deep bags work well for hand luggage and fast touch-ups; fold-out bags are most convenient at hotels.)

You can save space if you use a series of small makeup kits—one for hair, one for nails, one for your face, one for the body—and stuff them into shoes packed at the bottom of your suitcase. Of course, this means getting at the kits in flight is out of the question, so be sure to carry some cosmetics in your bag.

Pack your handbag. Include facial moisturizer and hand cream (tubes are best to avoid leaking), nondrying cleansing tissues, eye drops, washing solution for contact lenses or glasses, toothbrush, dental floss, toothpaste or powder, mouthwash or spray, purse-size perfume, lipstick (a lip pencil works better than a brush for applying lipstick while traveling because it is more controllable in jouncing), powder, compact, blushes, shadows, and lip gloss to avoid chapping.

Preparing Yourself for the Trip

Hair

On the day of your trip wash and condition your hair just the way you normally do, using products that suit your hair texture. The conditioner will coat each strand with a protective moisture seal to minimize high-altitude dryness and protect against broken and split ends.

Skin

You can partially protect your skin from excessive drying by taking a few extra minutes to follow this procedure before dressing to go to the airport.

1. Boil a small (about one-quart) saucepan of water.
2. Remove the pot from the heat and, draping a towel over your head and the pot to form a tent, allow the hot water vapors to circulate around your skin. Between ten and fifteen minutes under your little steam tent is usually sufficient to make your skin soft and moist.
3. Pat dry and then apply a moisturizer. I like Moisturel (Westwood); it has a nice consistency and is very good for dry skin.

Frantic last-minute rushes to the gate take their toll on your image. You may also find yourself in a sweat from carrying heavy bags. Before leaving home, use an antiperspirant or a combination product rather than a simple deodorant for sufficient protection in a stress-triggered situation.

Makeup

This is a good time to use a cream-base makeup, even if you usually use a liquid foundation. The oily base of the cream will act to guard your skin against moisture evaporation.

Use a cream blusher, creamy lipstick, and gloss on your lips for further protection. For flying, moist creamy eye shadows are preferable to powder shadows because they contain more oil.

The most annoying skin problem for most people on jet flights is the severe dehydration that leaves your hair brittle and your skin feeling dry and papery. Humidity in plane cabins is only 2 percent. The rate of evaporation aloft is 40 to 50 percent higher than at the same temperature at sea level. Moisturizing is a must. If countermeasures are not taken, your body can lose up to a quart more water in a single day of flying than it loses in a normal day on land. Don't leave home without your moisturizer; carry a small tube or jar with you. Apply it often to your throat, eye area, and the backs of your hands.

Lips and Eyes

Dehydration also affects your lips and eyes. Many travelers carry eye drops with them and use them from time to time. Drops moisten the eyes, lubricate them, and enhance your own protective tear fluid. Here are some products that work. All can be used by hard contact lens wearers:

- Tears Naturale (Alcon Labs)
- Liquifilm Tears (Allergan)
- Refresh (Allergan)—comes in disposable dispensers

Coat your lips with a lip balm or petroleum jelly. Try to avoid licking your lips, as that can increase the rate of moisture evaporation.

In-Flight Adjustments

How Dry I Am . . .

The first sign of discomfort aloft is usually dryness of your lips and eyes. They become irritated by the very low humidity in the airplane cabin and become dehydrated, along with the rest of your body and skin. This is a good time to reapply your moisturizer and a lip balm.

The dryness of plane cabins may be one reason why so many otherwise temperate passengers start ordering drinks even before the plane backs away from the gate. *Bad news:* Any alcohol, even wine, taken with your airline-prepared meals simply adds to the dehydration you are already experiencing. It also destroys the B vitamins that your body needs and has a direct negative effect on the air pressure discomfort that affects many passengers' ears when the plane descends. One drink aloft equals three at sea level and post-flight hangover lasts longer.

Carbonated beverages should be avoided, too, since the gases in them tend to expand in your intestines as a result of cabin pressures lower than those on land. I always pass on the liquors and sodas and ask for orange juice or mineral water, which contains calcium that facilitates nerve function and increases oxygen absorption.

Food of Flying

Eating lightly while you travel will make you more comfortable both during and after the trip; heavy food contributes to fatigue and stress. Leave sumptuous feasts for your return to earth. Take a tip from professional models and call ahead to order a fresh vegetable tray or a vegetarian meal. Crispy vegetables and fruits are loaded with needed vitamins and minerals and require less of your body's precious oxygen to digest. Foods heavy with protein, like steak and lobster, require oxygen for digestion and cause you to feel sleepy and less alert after eating.

Skin Bruises

You may find you sustain bruises and black and blue marks on your arms, legs, or body in the course of a flight. They are from bumps too slight to be noticed, such as lurching against a seat as you go to the rest room on the plane, or bumping against your own luggage. Your capillaries are under strain during flight; be gentle when washing your face or touching your skin in any way.

Ease Aloft

Once on your flight, you can take some further steps to ease the wearing effect of travel.

Sit in the nonsmoking section of the plane to save your skin. Nicotine, whether inhaled from your own cigarette or breathed in from someone else's cigarette, is irritating to your eyes, nose, and other mucous tissues. Carbon monoxide, a component of smoke, causes sluggishness.

In-Flight Exercises to Relieve Swelling and Puffiness

Here are some discreet exercises (movements) you can do while in your seat:

- *Legs:* Kick off your shoes and raise your feet so that they are almost level with your seat, just as you used to do as a child in your neighborhood movie theater. Rotate your ankles and curl and wiggle your toes. Hold your feet up for the count of ten, then relax. Repeat every half hour. (The grouch in the seat next to you may think you odd, but does that really matter? On really long flights everyone is squirming about anyway, so no one will question what you are doing.)
- *Shoulders:* Alternately raise each shoulder to the level of your ear, hold for the count of five, and relax. Next try to touch your elbows against the middle of your back. Hold for the count of five and relax.
- *Arms:* Reach up as high as possible, as if to turn on your overhead reading light; clasp your hands and turn your hands inside out, pulling the muscles of your arms and shoulders as much as possible.
- *Neck:* Loll your head forward and backward, then rotate it. (Do not do this if you suffer from motion sickness.)
- *Back and hips:* Balancing yourself on your hands, raise your body off the seat and hold for the count of five. Relax; repeat several times.

Swelling is another problem encountered by the traveler; it results from poor blood circulation on long trips. Your hands, feet, and ankles are affected the most. Wear loose-fitting clothes and shoes for maximum comfort. Wearing open-toed shoes on the day of the flight or thick socks or slippers on the plane also helps.

Relieving Jet Lag

Most people suffer more from jet lag when flying west to east than east to west, since getting up early is more challenging than lolling longer in bed. (Some people need as long as eighteen days to recover from a long eastbound flight.) People have specific biological time clocks that control the amount of hormones and blood chemicals released within their bodies at various times of the day, and flying eastward carries you counter to the path of the rotation of the earth and the pattern of light and sun you are used to. These changes, as well as the changes in local time and your body's time, can disrupt the body's carefully balanced rhythms and put you out of sync with your environment.

To minimize jet lag, choose your flight times carefully. Try to begin long trips in the morning hours to make adjustments easier. When you arrive, allow yourself an hour or two to reclaim your senses. Thanks to jet lag, bad moods may be the aftermath of any long flight, however thoughtful the cabin attendants.

Eating lightly and exercising a lot after your flight is over can help. Check into your hotel room, wash up, and make a plan. If the sun is still out, go for a walk or a jog; if night has fallen and local people are eating dinner, do some calisthenics in your room, then have a modest but nutritious meal as your dinner, even if at home you would now be having breakfast or lunch. Try to go to bed close to your normal hour based on local time, no matter what time it happens to be at home. A recent theory suggests that exposure to outdoor light helps accelerate adjustment to a new time zone.

Revival Tips

Often if I am traveling to a dermatological convention I have to attend a party on the day of my arrival. The following routine has helped me restore my energy and looks upon arrival at a hotel:

1. Take a relaxing bath.
2. If there is time, try to take a catnap.
3. Once awake, place chamomile teabags in cold water, then use them as compresses for your eyes.
4. Give yourself a refreshing facial with a mask.
5. If you still are lagged, place ice cubes on your wrists for a few moments.

At Your Destination

Feet Are Important

When you travel, take care of your feet. Your primary mode of transportation may be by plane, car, or boat, but a foot problem can prevent you from enjoying your trip and perhaps from going anywhere at all once at your destination. Carrying luggage strains your entire body, including your feet. Blisters develop easily as you slog along endless airport corridors. If you are prone to them, wear your shoes at home before the trip to be sure they fit comfortably. Never wear brand-new shoes. Wearing open-toed and open-heeled shoes helps prevent blisters. If you still develop a blister, cover it with a Band-Aid.

Tropical Treatment

Jetting to the Caribbean or Florida may sooth your chilblains, but the quick change to warmer weather will also stimulate the skin's sebaceous (oil) glands. The added oil and increased perspiration from warmer temperatures often combine to cause acnelike lesions. To prevent this problem, wash at least twice a day using the cleanser or soap you brought from home. (Be sure it is not a deodorant or antibacterial soap—these can react with the sunlight and cause a rash or sunburn.) Using scrubbing grains such as Clinique's Exfoliating Scrub or exfoliating pads such as Buf-Puf Singles (Personal Care Products/3M) will also help.

Rinse well, making sure to remove all traces of residue that would otherwise clog the pores. Apply an astringent (such as Sebanil/Owen or any alcohol solution, even cologne) with a water-soaked pad every morning to clear away dead skin cells and remove excess oil, thus making the pores appear smaller. To freshen up during the day, apply a few pats of chilled mineral water (put it in a spray bottle for a refreshing spritz).

In warm, sunny climates women should use slightly less makeup than usual and should switch to a water-based, oil-free brand. Do not cut out makeup altogether, however, because the pigments and colorants provide some sun protection. The best choice in warm weather makeup is a product that contains a sunscreen.

If you are headed toward a desert convention, meeting, or holiday, be forewarned that dry winds can dehydrate you rapidly, causing fatigue and listlessness. The Santa Ana winds of southern California and Arizona and similar dry winds can bring on headaches and irritability.

For an extended period in direct sunlight, choose powder blushes and lip pencils rather than creamy ones; powders are less likely to smear, because they have less oil in them. Pick a lipstick that contains sunscreen (a choice of several brands is available at most drugstores and cosmetic counters) or use a lip balm.

Food and Drink

Whether in the snow or warm sun, the exercise involved in outdoor sports leads to overheated muscles and potassium loss. This can bring on fatigue and muscle cramps, which are easily countered by eating potassium-rich fresh fruits. Oranges, melons, bananas, grapefruit, and pears are especially good to stave off problems and keep up energy and stamina (see chapter 17 for more about potassium).

The characteristic fruits of the tropics are very tempting, but you might find some of them bring along unpleasant surprises. The oily rind of the mango can cause swelling and an itchy rash similar to the reaction provoked by poison ivy, sumac, or oak. If you have allergies or are highly sensitive, use new plants and foods with caution. Even Hawaiian leis have been known to cause contact dermatitis.

When you have to drink the local water and can't boil it, add halazone tablets (available at your local pharmacy) to a quart of water and mix well. Store it for drinking and brushing teeth.

Beware of Local Animal Life

The local fauna should be treated with respect: Jellyfish and sea urchins, for example, often sting the unsuspecting vacation swimmer, causing a burning sensation and itchy welts. Touching or stepping on a spiny sea creature can cause painful punctures and splinter-like wounds. Mild over-the-counter antihistamines such as Chlor-Trimeton tablets can lessen these allergic reactions. (For more about bites and stings, see chapter 12.)

Dehydration—The Traveler's Biggest Skin Problem

When dehydration is your skin's problem, you can humidify yourself simply by running a tub of hot water and allowing it to steam you and everything else in your room for a while. Replace rapidly evaporating body fluids: Drink water, juices, and more water.

Altitude adjustment in mountain areas is hardest on those who smoke or have not exercised; slowing down just a bit can help. You cannot expect to perform at the same rate as you did at lower altitudes; less oxygen is available. That affects your thinking as well as your body. (Console yourself about the hardships of mountain living with the realization that because of the scarcity of oxygen, exercise at high altitudes burns off calories faster than at sea level.)

The problems your skin faces in the tropics or on icy mountain slopes are mostly minor annoyances if you exercise reasonable caution. Go ahead and enjoy your trip.

Bon Voyage

With simple forethought and planning, a woman can travel successfully anywhere in the world, knowing what to expect and how to manage intelligently—and she can do so with a sense of humor. Taking care of yourself is important everywhere, but especially when you are away from home. In case you are concerned about a possible need for medical assistance while away from home, Intermedic is an association that publishes an annual directory of hospitals where international travelers can reach English-speaking doctors. Membership is free. Write or call: Intermedic, 777 Third Avenue, New York, NY 10017; (212) 486-8900.

19

NINE TO FIVE... AND SOME WEEKENDS

Yes, I have career goals, just as you do. Women physicians are no different from other women, except we work extremely long hours. But you probably put in your share of eighty-hour weeks, too.

As women take advantage of broader career opportunities, employment-related skin problems keep pace. For women in business a skin problem is more than just an unpleasant irritation. Studies show that women are judged by their looks as well as performance. It is unfair, illegal, and even immoral, but it is true: Women who are more attractive usually earn more and have higher status.

Your job can irritate your skin. Most work-related skin problems come from two sources:

1. Irritants and allergens from the work environment or work materials can lead to allergic reactions.
2. Stress caused by anxiety, such as daily adjustments made in balancing a career and personal life—the not-enough-time syndrome—can affect skin and hair health.

Like many other aspects of life, some things can be changed, some controlled, and some avoided. I am endlessly vigilant for myself, and I always carefully question patients about their jobs. After all, a woman's skin, encompassing about 3,000 square inches, is her first line of defense against health-damaging infections. I often ask, "What kind of work do you do?" and "What materials do you handle?"

Recently a dramatic and attractive mature woman came to me for the first time. Her hands were red and scaly. She worked as an art curator for a well-known gallery. Only under questioning did she reveal that she had recently helped in restoring a series of old prints. After some detective work, I discovered that her skin was reacting to the solvents and glues used in her work. Although she had used solvents before, new formulas included somewhat different chemicals. Knowing about her allergy now helps her protect her skin.

Contact Dermatitis

Dermatitis means "inflammation of the skin." It is a disorder that often starts with itchy redness and swelling and can become severe enough to form blisters, oozing, and crusting. In chronic cases the skin becomes thickened, darkened, dry, and cracked.

When skin is directly exposed to harsh acids, alkalis, or other harmful agents for long enough (long enough may be briefly and just once) and in the right concentration (which may be just a touch), contact dermatitis can be the result.

An allergic reaction occurs when you make contact with an allergen and you become sensitized, or allergic, to that substance. That reaction can occur anywhere from a few days to a week or longer after initial contact with the sensitizing material. The rash can be widespread, not just at the point of contact. In the case of irritant contact dermatitis, a rash may appear almost immediately after contact at the site of the contact. No one can know if she is allergic to any substance until *after* she has a reaction.

Occupational Irritants and Allergens

Your office or workplace may be fraught with irritants and allergens. Your skin is your major contact with the environment and therefore often the first site of a reaction. Although chemicals cause over 90 percent of all industrial allergic reactions, finding an offending substance often takes patient detective work. Skin reacts to intrusions in a variety of ways— rashes, blemishes, redness, itching—which occur either immediately or after an unspecified time.

Some of the Triggers

Natural materials and synthetic resins are the most common sources of occupational skin problems, but almost anything can be the offending agent. The possible triggers are endless: Nickel, rubber, and hair dyes are the most common. A dedicated woman police officer found that she was allergic to the nickel in handcuffs—"making a collar" meant triggering a rash. Some other materials and situations that have been implicated follow.

Factors That Affect Allergic or Irritant Reactions

- *Gender:* Women are more sensitive than men to many irritants because their skin tends to be thinner and less oily then men's. (One Swedish study showed that 10 percent of women had allergic dermatitis, while only 2 percent of men were affected.)
- *Age:* Younger skin tends to be more sensitive than older skin; older skin inflames less easily.
- *Nutrition:* Faulty nutrition can be implicated in a skin reaction.
- *Stress*—certainly not unknown to working women
- *Emotions:* The range of moods on a busy day can affect allergic reactions.
- *Heredity:* Allergies or a predisposition to them can be inherited. Those with a personal or family history of atopy (hay fever, bronchial asthma) are more susceptible to skin reactions.

Friction

Pressure, even mild friction if repetitive, can act as an irritant. The rubbing of a substance against the skin, especially moist skin, can exacerbate or stimulate an allergic reaction. For example, a nickel or nickel alloy allergy (found in 10 percent of women) that might not usually cause a problem can flare up when fingers repeatedly rub against:

Tools	Dials	Door knobs	Cutlery
Coins	Paper clips	Letter openers	Buttons
Pots	Watchbands	Zippers	Snaps

Do your fingers itch after using that elegant metal letter opener? Are there small blisters on your fingers after you spend the day using the scissors? Both of these can indicate a nickel allergy. If you know that you are nickel sensitive, beware of objects that contain nickel, among them some jewelry, kitchen utensils, even detergents. A dermatologist can test you for nickel allergy and warn you of related allergies.

Several years ago a few of my jeans-wearing patients were bothered with irritations near the navel. It was a reaction to a metal stud on the waist button rubbing against the skin. The same sort of reaction can be triggered by plastic or rubber products, including rubber bands, pads, or gloves (rubber gloves used as protection can themselves be the source of the problem).

Product Coatings and Glues

Repeated handling of Oriental products coated with Japanese lacquer, a substance made from the Japanese lacquer tree, can bring on a reaction very similar to poison ivy, as can food handlers' contact with cashew nuts and mango skins. Plastics or other coatings are known irritants. Epoxy resins (commonly used in adhesives and on beer cans), glues, and insulating materials have also been implicated in rashes.

Environmental Factors

Extreme heat, humidity, dry air, wind, and rapid evaporation can bring out sensitivities. Exposure to X rays or other radiation also makes you more vulnerable. Bad lighting, high noise levels, and a poor quality of air in any work area can add to normal stress and affect reactions.

Plants

The most obvious of all sensitizing plants is poison ivy, but flowers and houseplants that are used as office decoration can cause skin problems, too. So can the mites in them and herbicides used on them. Plants known to cause an allergic reaction include:

Begonia	Yellow jasmine	Lilac
Sunflower	Ivy	Primrose
Daffodil	Aster	Chrysanthemum

Biological Invaders

Insects, bacteria, fungi, molds, yeast, and viruses are all around us all the time. Animal products such as lanolin, wool, and fur can also provoke reactions, and you certainly do not have to be a veterinarian for contact. An allergy to leather is common. If a sweater or jacket makes you feel itchy, do not wear it. Pure cotton garments are seldom irritating. In many cases the cause is not the fabric itself but a dye used to color it.

Chemicals

Although there are thousands of chemicals and chemical compounds, government workplace standards exist for a scant 600. Chemicals, especially alkalis in strong disinfectants and cleansers, destroy the skin's mildly acid mantle; acids burn the skin's surface. Chemicals and chemical compounds are sources of problems for food, laboratory, and medical workers, and for other "wet work" occupations.

Chemicals in cleansers, paints, solvents, etc., can also be the cause of allergy. While some chemicals may not result in irritation directly, on continued exposure they make skin more susceptible to damage through other means. Remove chemicals from clothing by dry cleaning or washing a few times in water to which a cup of vinegar has been added.

Cosmetics and Medicines

Parabens are used in the cosmetic industry as bacteria and fungi killers and have been known to cause occasional allergic reactions. Antihistamines, anesthetics, and antibiotics (especially neomycin) applied to the skin sometimes cause a reaction. In some cases dyes present in soaps can cause an allergic reaction of redness and swelling of the face and neck.

The Paper Chase

Paperwork, the bane of modern communications, carries irritants as well as information. The friction of handling papers can be irritating to the skin. In addition, formaldehyde and organic compounds found in duplicating fluids have been known to cause rashes. Other familiar office items that contain irritants and allergens are typewriter ribbons, stationery, Liquid Paper, carbon paper, and carbonless copy paper (NCR).

Irritants clinging to hands or fingers can be carried to the eyes. Abietic acid used in office paper has been found to cause a form of dermatitis similar to eczema, and multilith paper that contains sodium sulfonated naphthalene condensate also causes allergic reactions. Modern additions to offices, computers and word processors, bring a new potential for allergic reactions with their plastic housings and keyboards.

Several studies of the short- and long-term effects of computer video display terminals (VDTs) indicate there may be other problems with high technology (rashes on the face, redness and dryness of hands and forearms). Although it is too early for long-range conclusions, if you have allergies you are in a high risk category and should carefully consider those when weighing career options. Some jobs literally can make your skin sick.

How to Avoid Reactions

Many occupational skin reactions can be avoided by those with extremely sensitive skin if they wear clothing that covers the contact points, and if they use gloves or contact guards, such as cloth covers or cloth tape on dials. Cotton gloves are good protection. You can also use ordinary adhesive tape to cover certain tools or utensils. Wear protective gloves when handling chemicals or solvents and when gardening. The most practical way of avoiding further problems is washing your hands carefully to avoid spreading allergens and then coating your hands with a thin film of cream or other protective emollient. If your hands tend to peel and crack, use Gauz tape (a thin rubberized tape that provides a nonocclusive protective layer) to avoid additional trauma, even if it is only contact with papers.

Signs of trouble can be anything from dry, itchy skin to tiny blisterlike dots that appear on the fingers, especially on the finger sides. Some office skin sensitivities go untreated and are recognized only as a continuous minor annoyance until vacation time—when they miraculously disappear.

Occupational Acnes

If you are a chef or have another hot and greasy job, you have a good chance of developing acne from hot greases in the air of commercial kitchens. Fans circulate the air, so be sure a good ventilation system is installed and operating before you take any food-related position. Other jobs may also expose you to acne risks.

Chloracne

The severest of all occupational acne occurs in workers exposed to chemicals such as the chlorinated hydrocarbons and dioxin. These chemicals are included in pesticides and in hundreds of other chemical compounds. The acne triggered by these chemicals is called chloracne and is characterized by inflamed acne lesions and cysts on the face and body, which appear anywhere from two weeks to two years after exposure and may persist for years.

Initially the condition is mild: blackheads only, then whiteheads, and later yellowish cysts that resolve and leave dry, rough patches.

In severe cases, there is a swelling of the upper eyelids and darkening of the skin and conjunctiva. Typically the victims suffer cysts under the arms and in the groin area as well as on the cheeks; the nose is usually spared. Workers of all ages and both sexes are equally vulnerable. Chloracne is generally resistant to conventional acne therapy, though Accutane has been used successfully.

Anyone working in or near a chemical plant should exercise extreme care: Minute traces of offending substances can cause chloracne. Disregarding any rash, flare-up of blemishes, itching, or swelling is a mistake. You cannot tell whether or not you are susceptible until you see some sign of a problem. Vigilance is vital.

Businesswoman's Acne

Imagine a busy, bright young perfectionist—a professional woman, middle manager, or entrepreneur. She probably takes or has just stopped taking birth control pills. Go further: Imagine that she moves and eats quickly at restaurants and often selects shellfish because it is low in calories and high in protein. She is fond of red wine. Although she uses makeup, she is too busy to spend more than a few minutes washing and rinsing her face. You are imagining a woman courting adult acne. Adult acne is often recognized as:

- Fast-track acne—a reaction to stress from self-induced or from external forces
- Acne rosacea—heredity, personality, and skin type set the stage, but a tough competitive workplace can trigger this acnelike condition.
- Pill acne—triggered by birth control pills
- Medication acne—a side effect of prescription and over-the-counter medications that keep you going when you just can't take a day off
- Food acne—the result of a high androgen content in foods that commonly comprise quick take-out lunches, of long luncheon meetings with the wrong menu, and of some health foods that affect the skin

- Cosmetic acne—more likely the result of incorrect cleansing than of any makeup

(See chapter 5 for more information about why grown women suffer acne flareups.)

Makeup at Work

What you want from an office makeup may be somewhat different from what is needed from a sports makeup or a social evening's makeup. At work, women want reliability and longevity more than drama.

The right makeup protects your skin. Makeup can add years to your professional life. Women who have worn makeup for several years often have smoother, clearer, firmer, and younger-looking skin than their more "natural" sisters. The oils in cosmetics delay the evaporation of moisture from the skin, and the pigments in cosmetics act as a partial barrier against ultraviolet rays from sun and artificial lighting. Correct application and removal techniques allow you to use makeup and have clear skin, too. New trends in cosmetics make good-for-you makeup possible for almost everyone.

The Working Woman's Basics in Choosing Makeup

- Start by selecting a light, watery moisturizer such as:
      Keri Light (Westwood)
      Neutrogena Moisture (Neutrogena)
      Nutraderm (Owen)
- Wear a sunscreen makeup or sunscreen under your makeup if you work under fluorescent lights, because fluorescent light bulbs emit ultraviolet A light. (The amount of UVA exposure received by an office worker from fluorescent lights during a one-year period equals the amount received in forty minutes of outdoor exposure.)
- Indoor workers who have any tendency toward acne should check the labels to be sure that a moisturizer is low in oils and other comedogenic ingredients.
- Outdoor workers need protection in the form of a heavier moisturizer, but do not overdo the moisturizing—and add a UVA/UVB protecting sunscreen. In hot weather skip the moisturizer. (For more advice about outdoor protection, see chapter 12.)
- Mascara and eye shadow reduce glare from video display terminals or shiny substances.

Basics in Applying Your Working Makeup

- If you have a tendency to small bumps in the skin, use a water-based foundation. Surprisingly, pancake products that are applied with a damp sponge have good coverage, last through daylong meetings, and seldom cause trouble. (Max Factor's Pancake Makeup is a good example.)
- Avoid applying new makeup over old makeup; the new coat of foundation will capture dirt, perspiration, and oils on the skin's surface.
- Loose powders, especially cornsilk powders that have a high proportion of cornstarch in them, are preferable to pressed powders for touchups because they absorb facial oils.

How to Wash Your Face at Work

The right makeup is important, but removing it thoroughly is even more important.

The key to keeping smooth, attractive skin and well-groomed hair is cleanliness. Cleansing washes away stress-stimulated oils from the pores and microorganisms and allergens from the skin's surface, as well as dust, dirt, and dead cells.

Avoid scrubbing or any vigorous handling—the less stimulation of the skin, the better. Zip through anything else, but be sure that every smidgin of debris or residue is off your face. Rinse with cool water to tighten pores.

Air-dry or gently pat dry your skin. Never scrub with rough paper towels or use the communal cloth towels that are provided in some washrooms. Moist skin is easily irritated and more vulnerable to infections than dry skin. To be absolutely clean, you can use a mild freshener or toner to make pores seem smaller and tighter. For dry skin, dilute the freshener by applying with a water-soaked cotton ball or pad. Do not use an astringent near the eyes or throat area.

The physical activity of washing your face midday at work can alleviate some stress and give you the added bonus of looking fresher for the afternoon. The act of bending, lathering, rinsing, etc., changes your circulation and brings a fresh blood supply to your face.

For touch-ups carry a natural or man-made sponge that can be moistened under cold water and applied to your face, or apply a cold moistened paper towel to your face. It will cool the skin and slow oil production. Dry skin can also be helped by applying moisture on the surface, and then smoothing on moisturizer as needed.

If getting to water to wash your face is a problem or you are short on time, use Take Off (Personal Products Company) tissues for cleansing.

Hands and Nails at Work

Even a businesswoman's hands are exposed to a great deal of day-to-day abuse. Just the number of times you wash and dry your hands—and how you do it—can affect your skin and nails.

How to Wash Your Hands at Work Without Irritating Your Skin

Follow these seven steps to avoid problems:

1. Remove all your rings before washing. Jewelry can trap irritating material and even lead to hand dermatitis.
2. Use lukewarm rather than hot water.
3. Use as little and as mild a soap as necessary; more will not do a better cleaning job but can irritate your skin.
4. Do not scrub; stroke gently, gliding the soap or lather on the surface of the palms. Avoid rubbing soap into the backs of the hands.
5. Avoid the alkaline soaps and detergents that are supplied in most workplace bathrooms or in public buildings. They can aggravate other skin problems and lead to chapping and irritations. Bring your own soap with you, if it is convenient. If you routinely need to wash hands often, as I do, you might try using a mild facial cleanser such as Neutrogena's or Crabtree & Evelyn's, which both come in a pump bottle.
6. Rinse soap off thoroughly.
7. Pat your hands dry before applying a nonoily moisturizer such as:
   Lubriderm Lotion (Warner-Lambert)
   Carmol-10 Lotion (Syntex)
   New Formula Complex-15 Hand Lotion (Baker/Cummins)
   Lacticare Lotion (Stiefel)

If your workplace bathroom does not have hand towels but uses a hot-air blower to dry hands, bring a towel from home. Hot-air blowers have been associated with chapped hands. If you must use the hot-air blower, keep your hands at least six inches from the nozzle and dry your hands thoroughly.

Nail Flicking and Other Nail Breakers

As noted in chapter 16, typing and drumming of the nails seem to make them grow stronger and faster. (Think of harpists, guitarists, and other strong-nailed musicians.) But nail flicking—bending the nail of one finger with another nail—may cause the disruption of fine blood vessels in the nail bed. Little streaks of pink or red appearing near the tip of the nail are a sign of this.

Nervously picking hangnails, those triangular-shaped pieces of hard skin that form over the sides and cuticle edges of the nails, and biting nails are nail-damaging habits. Some commonsense advice:

- Clip these hangnails and try not to pick them.
- Dial telephones with a dialer or switch to a button phone.
- Do not pick up small objects with your nails—use the pads of your fingers.
- Wear gloves when outside in cold weather—nails can become damaged.
- Rub your hand lotion well into the flesh surrounding your nails to keep the area soft. New Formula Complex-15 Hand Cream or Lotion (Baker/Cummins) has been reported to actually strengthen nails.

Wet Work

If you wash your hands often, submerge your hands in water, or allow your hands to remain moist for long periods of time, the skin becomes vulnerable to infections. Hand dermatitis is common among those who do wet work. Be aware, too, that those with hand dermatitis are more prone to nickel allergy.

People in occupations that require washing several times an hour (doctors and other medical personnel, housewives, cooks) can easily contract paronychia, an annoying fungal infection. Bartenders and waitresses who handle beer, which is yeasty, are particularly susceptible. When the infection strikes the nail fold, the fold becomes red and swollen; the nail loses its luster, becomes greenish, and develops transverse or longitudinal ridges. Very severe cases of infection result in red, moist, white-centered patches between the fingers, most often between the third and ring fingers.

If you cannot get away from moisture or wet work, even for a short time, you can resort to wearing waterproof rubber or plastic gloves with cotton liners or over separate cotton gloves (sold as beauty or cosmetic gloves). I recommend having a few dozen pairs of cotton gloves and switching them every half hour when you are doing wet work. Overexposure to detergents and hot water can cause soft nails.

Many nail problems can be averted by wearing gloves. But wearing rubber gloves alone for long periods can trap hand perspiration inside the gloves, creating irritation and increasing the chance of an infection. Some women find that sprinkling talcum powder inside their gloves is helpful.

Nails Discolored by Work

Discolored nails are fairly common. Some physicians can guess your occupation by the specific discoloration of your nails:

- Work with chemicals such as pesticides and chromium salts—or with flowers—has a tendency to turn nails yellow.
- Gray or bluish nails are seen on photographers, textile workers, and those who handle silver or gold.

- Photographers, bakers, and cooks can have brownish nails.
- Green nails are common among restaurant and bar employees, house-keepers, and housewives.

Polish Protects

Nail polish can actually protect and even strengthen nails. If you do not like bright or deep shades, use light or clear polish. Always use a base coat so your manicure will last longer. It will also prevent your nails from yellowing due to absorption of the pigment in the nail enamel. Using Develop 10 (Vital Nails) as a top coat will prolong your manicure. Allow ample time for the polish to dry.

A carefully done manicure with a base and top coat should last a week or ten days, although light touch-ups might be necessary to repair cracks and chips. (For more about nails and a perfect manicure see chapter 16.)

Hair at Work

The same stresses that can trigger acne can cause hair loss. Thinning hair can start with an oily scalp and dandruff. Just as with skin, emotional overload can be a trigger factor.

Sometimes the need to look authoritative and professional can lead to hair-restricting styles such as ponytails, buns, braids, or excessive teasing, all of which can lead to permanent damage. Taut, confined hairstyles may be damaging to hair growth. Businesswomen tend to overhandle their hair, shampooing and styling it daily. Be sure to condition and deep-condition your hair regularly; try giving it a day off on the weekend. An instant shampoo for light-haired women in a bind: Try brushing talcum powder through your hair to absorb oil.

Do not wear a hat or hair covering if you work inside, and always wear a hat or hair covering if you work outdoors. Growing numbers of women are employed in hard-hat jobs. Hat weight can break hair, irritate the scalp by preventing perspiration from evaporating, and even suppress new hair growth. (For more about hair care see chapter 13.)

Working Women, Beware!

More than 55,000 occupations are listed by the federal government, and millions of women work inside and outside the home. These figures multiply into endless opportunities for women to achieve their career goals—and to run up against work-related skin problems. Caution and proper care mini-mize the problems and let the natural beauty of your skin, nails, and hair represent you at your best.

For more information about occupational skin safety write: Occupational Safety and Health Administration, U.S. Department of Labor, 200 Constitu-tion Avenue NW, Washington, D.C. 20210.

20

WHAT YOU NEED TO KNOW TO HAVE ALLURING EYES

I have noticed that even with the best medical help it can take several weeks to improve your complexion—but it usually takes only one sleepless night to make you look awful. Sleep is seldom thought of as one of the factors that affects the skin, but I see the difference between adequate rest and sleeplessness in my own looks and the looks of my patients as well.

Six Sleep-Ease Tips

The older we get, the less we sleep and the fewer dreams we have. Sleep or the lack of it dramatically affects how we look. The following sleep tips may help:

1. Your mattress should be eight to ten inches longer than your height and at least ten inches wider than your body at its widest part to allow for the twenty to fifty changes of position most of us make each night.
2. The heavier you are the firmer your mattress should be; very slender women with less natural padding will be more comfortable on a soft mattress.
3. Your pillow should be no fuller than the space between your head and shoulders. To test for pillow size, stand next to a wall and place the

pillow between your head and the wall; it should not force your head forward. Sleeping on your back without any pillow at all is most advantageous to the skin. You risk asymmetrical creases and wrinkles on the side of your face you like to sleep on when you lie on your side.

4. Natural fibers—silk, linen, wool, and cotton—are the best choices for bedding to avoid static electricity that comes from rubbing against synthetic fibers. Wool blankets can cause skin reactions in some people. (If you are sensitive to wool, avoid them.)

5. During sleep you breathe approximately thirty barrels of air; keep your windows open, if only just a crack.

6. The best sleep temperature is between 60° and 64°F. Lower temperatures will make you require more sleep to feel rested; higher temperatures will cause you to be restless during sleep. If the temperature is over 70°F, you may not sleep long enough.

Puffy Eyes—Causes and Remedies

Puffy morning eyes become common in the third or fourth decade of life. Fluid accumulation in the eye area, which leads to puffy eyes, can be triggered by a great range of factors:

Too much sleep	Crying
Cardiac failure	Overactive or underactive thyroid
A cold	Too little sleep
Vitamin C deficiency	Kidney problems
Sinus infections	Trauma
Stress	Allergic reactions

Raising your head slightly by placing two- to four-inch blocks of wood under the legs at the head of the bed can help, if you don't mind sleeping on a slant. Other methods to help avoid puffy eyes rely on changing some of your daily habits and routines:

- Stick to a low-sodium diet.
- Switch to another brand of eye cream. Try a light coating of petroleum jelly for several nights to see if your usual cream could be inspiring an allergic reaction and causing the problem.
- Avoid eye makeup for a few days. Eye makeup remover can also be at fault; try baby oil for removal if you cannot do without eye makeup.
- Be gentle. Dot and pat on all cosmetics—don't stroke or rub.
- Allergic reactions to mascara include itchy, tearing eyes and reddened, swollen skin around the eyes. If you have these symptoms, avoid the use of mascara long enough to determine if it is at fault.
- Don't drink any fluids less than thirty minutes before bedtime.

- Avoid alcoholic beverages, especially strong drinks or large quantities.
- Discontinue the use of any eye creams that include vitamin E. It is not entirely understood why, but many of them create puffy eyes.

To reduce puffiness, try salt compresses (one teaspoon of salt per glass of cool water).

Maintaining Youthful Eyes

The skin around your eyes is one of the first areas to show your age. The skin on the eyelids and under the eyes is very thin and very easily stretched. Nature placed thin skin here to permit the rapid eye movements necessary to protect your eyes. The skin around your eyes is unique in another way: It has modified sebaceous glands that, unlike the oil glands in other parts of the face or body, provide very little natural oil.

Age and heredity often conspire to make eyes look tired and "just woke up." The skin tone of your eye area depends on the strength and elasticity of collagen and elastin fibers, and that is an inherited factor, as is the shape of your skull and the orbits (eye sockets). As to why the effects of aging show up first around the eyes, the drier and thinner the skin covering the eye area, the more likely it is that your eyes will look older than you are. Use an eye cream such as Maximum Eye Care (Estée Lauder), Visible Difference Eye Care Concentrate (Elizabeth Arden), or one of the new eye creams with sunscreen added.

As you grow older the amount of support tissue around the eyes lessens. Fat, which lumps with age instead of staying in a soft, youthful pad, pushes out of the socket to create prominent fatty deposits and make the eyes look puffy and baggy.

If serious damage to the skin around your eyes is already evident, cosmetic surgery, either as part of a total facelift or in a separate procedure called a *blepharoplasty,* is the way to eliminate it. (More about blepharoplasty later in this chapter.)

Banishing Bags Under the Eyes

Until you are ready for surgery use cosmetics to minimize the problems. Carefully applied cosmetics can camouflage baggy eyes. Here is how to smooth a bag cosmetically:

1. Use a concealer one shade lighter than your skin (apply with a light sable brush).
2. Paint a light line from your inner eye corner along the base of the bag.
3. With the fourth finger of your hand, lightly tap the line, to blend it well.

Use the concealer over your foundation and use as little as possible. Don't powder; the powder will cake on the concealer. Avoid thick, waxy concealers that are hard to blend. Three products that have worked well for many women are Under Eye Over Cream (Almay), Erace (Max Factor), and Stage Ten Neutralizer (Stage Ten).

Dark Circles Under the Eyes

Almost every woman has noticed dark areas or circles under her eyes from time to time. They can appear for no apparent reason or they can be traced to a particular cause, such as a sleepless night. Many other factors can cause their appearance:

Thin skin. When the skin is extremely thin, the blood supply running under the skin is visible, showing through as dark bluish shadows. This is most evident in the eye area when the rest of the face is pale by contrast.

Pallor. If the circles under your eyes seem darker when you are tired or when you are indoors, you may just be noticing them more because of the pallor of your skin. Very probably exercise is what you need to make the rest of your face less pallid and to stimulate the circulation. You may also need a vacation.

Iron deficiency anemia. Dark circles can come from a mild form of iron deficiency anemia that can be cured by a change in your diet and more rest. Iron-rich food, fresh air, and exercise are probably all that are needed. (For more about iron deficiency anemia and a diet to counter it, see chapter 17.)

Menstruation. Circles under the eyes often signal the onset of menstruation. They are possibly the result of a change in the hormones of the body or due to the rapid loss of premenstrually retained liquids.

Melanin production. Dark circles can also be a product of melanin deposits in the skin beneath the eyes. Sunlight is the primary stimulant of melanin production, although stress can sometimes work the same way. The effect is often seen in severely ill persons as well as in the chronically tired and overworked. Using a sunblock on the area underneath the eyes and wearing protective sunglasses when you are in bright sunlight may help prevent this problem. Two sunblocks that will protect the eye area are Eye-Zone Sun Block (Clinique) and Bain de Soleil Under Eye Protector 15 (Charles of the Ritz). Of course, to undo the effects of severe chronic stress, you will need to reorganize your life. If you do, dark circles under your eyes won't be the only problem you will cure.

Rubbing. Stressing your eyes by frequent rubbing or pulling on the lids can lead to dark circles.

Heredity. Hyperpigmentation of the eyelids and under the eyes may be hereditary; it sometimes appears in childhood.

Dark circles can also be an indication of an endocrine problem or biliary duct disease or can be chemically induced. The use of certain eye ointments that contain mercury or silver compounds may produce permanent darkening and grayish brown lids.

Cosmetic Coverage for Dark Circles

Use cosmetics to make dark circles less obvious. The idea is to draw attention upward, away from the area under the eye.

1. Apply foundation under the eyes.
2. Then apply a very light orangish blusher over the area.
3. Use a gray or blue shadow and lots of mascara, but only on the upper lashes.

Hanging Skin Above the Eyes

The skin between the crease of the eyelids and the brows dries and loosens with age and can seem to hang over the eye. The loose skin is not only unattractive, it can cause eye fatigue and in extreme cases impair vision. Even just a bit of slack skin creates difficulty when you want to apply eye shadow and other eye makeup.

You can delay problems of this type by preserving moisture within the skin. Smooth oil over the area whenever possible to hold moisture in. Eye shadows protect the skin and can serve as a barrier against sun damage, but removing the shadow with vigorous rubbing can be worse than using no shadow at all. Always lubricate the area and then blot the pigments and the oil away. Don't wipe, stretch, or stroke the skin in any way.

Here are two safe commercial eye makeup removers:

- Extremely Gentle Eye Makeup Remover (Clinique)
- Effacil Gentle Eye Makeup Remover (Lancôme)

Wide-Open, Youthful Eyes

Here's how to use makeup to correct the problem of drooping eyelids:

1. Apply your eyeliner over the drooping lid.
2. Draw a straight line on the lower eyelid.
3. Shade the area just under the eyebrow with a light tone to draw attention upward to the brow.

If your eyelid has the slightest tendency to droop, hold the weak, loose tissue with your fingers when you apply makeup.

Blepharoplasty (Cosmetic Surgery)

Little can be done at home to improve drooping eyelids once the elastic tissue has weakened. When extra skin is observable on the lids, it is time to consider blepharoplasty. This procedure is done by a cosmetic plastic surgeon and can be very successful.

The surgeon will first carefully examine your lids, vision, and eye motions, take careful measurements and perhaps photographs in preparation. Using local anesthesia, the surgeon removes the excess skin from the upper eyelid and removes fat-containing compartments in other areas around the eye. Cold compresses are applied to the eyes right after surgery to minimize bleeding and swelling. Laughing and vigorous chewing should be avoided for about three days. However, when the stitches come out on the fourth day, makeup and mascara can be used.

Eyes Right

To keep your eyes clear avoid eyestrain, too much computer programming, cigarette smoke, the common cold, and sensitizing (allergy producing) materials. Remember that the redness of irritated eyes is a signal to change something you're doing, not just to medicate the symptoms away.

21

MOTHERHOOD
AND YOUR LOOKS

When you are pregnant, you experience the most dramatic and exciting body changes that will ever affect the way you look and feel. The major changes in your silhouette will be accompanied by important changes in your hair, nails, and skin.

Hormonal Changes

The glow of pregnancy has physiological as well as emotional causes. Hormonal and vascular changes such as the elevated estrogen level and increased circulation are responsible. The inner changes are generally reflected externally in a new radiance by the fourth or fifth month.

The physiological changes of the skin that occur during pregnancy are to a great extent triggered by changes of hormones within the body.

Many women look better when pregnant than at any other time of their lives. Pregnancy brings on many hormonal changes, particularly an increase in the amount of female sex hormones that are present. Estrogen levels rise around the seventh to tenth week of pregnancy, and changes in skin texture, tone, and color usually follow. The increase in estrogen during pregnancy has been linked with feelings of calm and well-being. There is also a lowered risk of mental illness during this time.

Progesterone, another hormone, is produced by the placenta; the percentage of this hormone in the body during pregnancy is ten times greater than before pregnancy. It is thought that this hormone also has a calming effect; a study done at the Stanford Medical School indicated that it brought relief from depression.

All that good feeling has a very positive effect on your looks as well as your disposition. The added estrogen also makes your skin soft and glowing and your hair thicker than normal.

Skin Color Changes When Pregnant

Ninety percent of all pregnant women notice a change in the color of their skin—it becomes slightly darker. They need to use a makeup foundation and other cosmetics that are a shade or two deeper than their usual shade.

Here is where you can expect color changes when pregnant:

- The lips and genital area often become noticeably deeper in shade and purplish or even bluish in cast; nipples and areolae (areas around the nipples) usually become darker.
- Scars, freckles, and other already dark areas such as the armpits, the crook of the elbow, and the areas behind the knees darken further.
- The line of connective tissue called the linea alba (a white line) that runs along the middle of the abdomen from the chest to the pubic area darkens. It is then called the linea nigra, a black line.

Most of these changes remain throughout pregnancy and will fade only three or four months after delivery. However, the darker your skin is to start with, the greater the chance that hyperpigmentation will last.

Melasma—The Mask of Pregnancy

The most prevalent and cosmetically unpleasant side effect of pregnancy is a blotchy pigmentation on the face called melasma.

Although my mother did not suffer melasma when she was carrying me, I was so concerned about melasma that I bought a large wide-brimmed hat to wear during my pregnancy. I started wearing it early in the spring and continued to wear hats until the delivery.

Melasma appears as large tan or brown spots or patches that have irregular borders and are arranged in a netlike pattern on the face—around the eyes, and on the cheeks, upper lip, forehead, chin—and neck. The area around the eyes and above the brows becomes masklike in severe cases, winning malasma notoriety as "the mask of pregnancy." This darkening affects over 70 percent of all pregnant women and ranges in intensity from faint to disfiguring. Melasma is more noticeable on dark-skinned women. (Birth control pills can cause a hint of melasma; if you developed this discoloration while on the pill, take extra care during pregnancy.)

How Your Doctor Tests for Melasma

The discolorations of melasma are caused by melanin deposits, possibly in different levels of your skin. When your dermatologist studies your skin under a Wood's light (an ultraviolet light source fitted with a cobalt filter that is used to diagnose skin conditions), the depth or level of discoloration will be evident. The depth of the discoloration determines your dermatologist's choice of treatment. The more superficial the melanin deposits, the more likely it is the condition will respond to bleaching creams.

In normal daylight melasma may look mottled or spotted—the discolored areas seem to blend with the normal skin. More often they form distinct areas with sharp edges.

Weather Guards Against Melasma

The sun promotes and amplifies any skin discoloration, even a hormonally triggered one: Dark areas of the skin deepen even more when exposed to the sunlight. Avoid any sunning and tanning when pregnant. A wide-brimmed hat should be part of your maternity wardrobe, and scarves and gloves help, too. Wind, low humidity, and other weather phenomena may also irritate and make skin look darker and blotchy, but those changes are usually temporary; the sun is the real culprit.

Sunscreens and sunblocks can retard or entirely prevent skin discoloration, especially those products with an SPF of 15 or higher. However, sunscreens containing PABA do not protect the skin from exposure to ultraviolet A rays, nor do they shield against photoreactions suffered with certain drugs. Use sunblocks regularly during pregnancy, regardless of the season. Use an opaque sunblock or a sunscreen with benzophenones and PABA. Here are some recommended products with high concentrations of titanium oxide:

- Solar Cream (Doak)
- Continuous Coverage (Clinique)
- Reflecta (Texas)
- RVPaque (Elder)

Sunblocks are good protection from melasma and sensible skin protectors against the aging effects of the sun's rays.

For maximum protection use as sunscreen under your makeup foundation and over any light moisturizer you might be wearing. Some moisturizers and foundations include a sunscreen in their formula. Try to use such products even in the middle of winter.

Besides a foundation with sunscreen, try to use blushers and other makeup colors that include a screen. The pigments in blushers, some powders, and some eye shadows actually provide protection to the skin by deflecting many of the sun's rays and preventing them from penetrating the skin deeply. (For more about avoiding the ultraviolet rays of the sun, see chapter 6.)

Bleaching Melasma—Reversing the Damage

Once the skin has been damaged and darkened by the sun, lightening it up again with bleaches is a long and difficult task. One of the most popular skin bleaches is a preparation containing hydroquinone. Used in freckle creams as well as bleaches, hydroquinone is slow acting and, in over-the-counter concentrations of 2 percent or less, practically useless. But it can work if you ask your doctor for a prescription of 3 percent or higher. However, note that prolonged usage of hydroquinone can turn fingernails brown.

It can take several months to fade discolorations and you might not see any improvement at all for about four to five weeks. Worst of all, one suntan can undo all your efforts; you can develop marked melasma in just a few days of unprotected sunning. If bleaching agents don't work, ask your dermatologist about electrodesiccation, chemical peels, and other such treatments in case your melasma does not disappear within six months after delivery. (For more about how to use skin bleaches and other treatments, see chapter 23.)

Broken Blood Vessels in the Face

During pregnancy, usually in the second to fifth month, women with thin, fair skin often notice small red lines appearing for the first time on and around the nose and inside the nostrils. These so-called broken capillaries (telangiectases) are the result of permanent dilation of tiny blood vessels near the surface of the skin. Nobody knows exactly what causes them, though high estrogen levels increase the number of visible small blood vessels, particularly in women with a predisposition to broken capillaries.

Avoiding Broken Capillaries

If even one of these dilated vessels appears (the nose is a favorite first site), you must:

- Avoid drinking any alcohol; alcohol dilates the blood vessels of the skin. (Pregnant women should avoid alcohol anyway, since more and more evidence now links alcohol to birth defects.)
- Avoid pressing, tugging, or fingering any part of the face. Hands off. Don't rest your face on your hands or pressure your skin in any way. Blows, bruises, and other trauma can also affect the small blood vessels near the surface of the skin.

If you have a tendency to broken blood vessels, wash your skin gently; avoid the use of beauty grains or scrubs, washcloths, and abrasive commercial pads.

Some medications, including niacin, can bring an unwanted flush to the skin. Be cautious about hot or spicy foods; chili, curry, and other overly seasoned foods can cause damage. Also avoid drinking very hot liquids. (For more about how to avoid and treat dilated blood vessels, see chapter 23.)

Spider Angiomas

Sometimes broken capillaries appear in the shape of a spider. These are called spider angiomas. About two-thirds of pregnant women get spider angiomas—one or several—most often on the face, especially around the eyes, but also on the neck, upper chest, hands, and arms. Most spider angiomas disappear within three months after the baby is born. If they don't go away by themselves, a dermatologist can remove them (the procedure is similar to the removal of telangiectases).

Help for Broken Capillaries

If you develop broken blood vessels on your face or elsewhere on your skin, something can be done about it. Your dermatologist can electrodesiccate, or seal off, a broken blood vessel. The sealing is done with an electric needle similar to the needle used in electrolysis. The doctor applies the needle to the red line and, without too much pain or discomfort, it disappears. Sometimes a few treatments are necessary, particularly for spider angiomas.

Once the vessel is sealed, blood can no longer flow through it, so the red line is no longer noticeable. It is actually blood flowing through the damaged, dilated tube that causes a visible red marking. Electrodesiccation takes very little time and is relatively inexpensive.

Varicose Veins

About 40 percent of pregnant women develop superficial (small) varicose veins commonly known as spider veins (I call them vanity veins). These are actually dilated capillaries. In general, varicose veins during pregnancy are caused by increased pressure within the large veins of the pelvis (due to the enlarged uterus), which makes it difficult for blood to flow back from the legs. Preexisting varicose veins are very likely to worsen during pregnancy. Women whose mothers had varicose veins are more likely to see varicose veins during their own pregnancies. Obesity also predisposes women to varicose veins during pregnancy.

Controlling Varicose Veins

Here are some ways to minimize the appearance of varicose veins during pregnancy:

- Keep legs elevated whenever possible.
- Avoid prolonged sitting or standing.
- Don't sit with legs crossed.

- Sleep with a pillow under your legs or with the bottom of the bed elevated.
- If you travel often, exercise on the plane to keep blood flowing.
- Wear support pantyhose or elastic stockings (Jobst or Sigvaris).
- Avoid wearing boots that grip the legs.
- Eat foods high in fiber.

Treatment of Varicose Veins

Sclerotherapy, injections of irritating solutions into the veins, is the most common treatment for spider veins. A number of solutions are available; I prefer a hypertonic (highly concentrated) solution of saline. This solution injected with a very fine needle directly into the veins is irritating enough to cause a gradual obliteration of the blood vessel. Irritation and subsequent inflammation of the injected vessel walls force the blood from the vessel and connecting branches, resulting in a permanent closure (sclerosis) of the vessel. If blood vessels can't carry blood, they can't be seen.

The technique is simple but requires precision. The results can be seen in a few weeks to a few months. A few treatments at two-week intervals are usually necessary; the number of treatments depends on the extent of the problem. The injections cause a mild burning sensation, and you may have some redness and swelling in the area or develop hives around the injection for a short time. Occasionally, postinjection pain occurs, most likely as a result of muscle spasm. This is not uncommon when spider veins around the ankles are injected. Darker skinned women can also develop brownish spots at the site of injection. Time will usually fade these, but a bleaching agent will accelerate the process. Immediately after injections, a woman can return to her regular activities.

These treatments should never be done during pregnancy—wait until after delivery. (During pregnancy you can camouflage the veins with coloring agents.) Treatment is also contraindicated if you are undergoing any type of hormonal treatment of if you have a history of phlebitis or pulmonary embolism.

Mottled Skin

High color, a tendency to vascular reactions, sensitive skin, and the added weight of pregnancy can bring on an unpleasant mottled—almost moiré or marbleized—finish to the skin whenever you are exposed to cold. The surface seems uneven in tone and slight areas of almost pinkish purple appear in different places, mostly the legs. The same effect can be seen on the skin of an infant, probably because the skin is so thin that the blood supply is almost visible beneath the surface. To avoid this effect, which is not harmful in itself, try to keep your temperature even; avoid dramatic changes between hot and cold that can make your skin change from flushed to pallid.

Skin Tags

Tiny flesh-colored growths of skin, usually no larger than a pencil point, can appear on your skin during pregnancy, usually toward the end. The cause for the growth of these tiny tags of skin, called *acrochordons,* is not really understood. They usually appear in groups, most often under the arms, on the neck, on the upper chest, or under the breasts. They are more of a nuisance than a reason to worry, although they can be frightening because they grow so rapidly. Happily, skin tags never become cancerous.

Most of the time skin tags disappear after the mother gives birth. If you find them irritating and disfiguring, however, you can ask your dermatologist to cut or burn them off. But it's best to postpone as much surgery as possible until after the delivery.

Stretch Marks

The longest lasting and most feared skin problem associated with pregnancy is stretch marks, which afflict about 90 percent of all pregnant women. These long rivers of lighter skin, technically called *striae distensae,* can appear anywhere but are most prevalent on the breasts, hips, flanks, and abdomen. They may also appear on the buttocks, groin, thighs, and upper arms. Stretch marks develop from a rapid distension of the skin that is beyond the elasticity of the elastic and collagen skin fibers to endure. They are common in pregnancy because the weight gain is so rapid—they usually become noticeable during the sixth month of gestation.

Here is the bad news: Once stretched too far, the skin can no longer resume its former condition. At present there is no way to remove stretch marks. Options are limited to cosmetic disguise.

During pregnancy, stretch marks tend to be pink, crimson, or purplish. Most women panic at their first appearance and rush for the cocoa butter (a folklore remedy), sap from an aloe plant, or vitamin E oil (more modern folklore), but to no avail.

Cosmetically, time heals more than any of these remedies. No amount of patting, oiling, brushing, stimulating, massaging, or hoping can make a difference.

Why Some Women Develop the Marks and Others Don't

If you are intent on avoiding stretch marks, avoid gaining weight rapidly, since a speedy weight gain at any time can stretch skin and rupture the elastic fibers. (Adolescents going through rapid body and weight changes are also prone to stretch marks.) Once you are pregnant, whether or not you get stretch marks depends mostly on heredity. Another factor possibly at work is fluctuation in the balance of certain hormones. Some medications (systemic steroids and salves and lotions that contain cortisone-like preparations) seem to provoke marks when used for long periods or under occlusive dressings. Further research on the subject is likely to follow.

Dealing with Stretch Marks

If you already have stretch marks, a surgeon can remove them. But keep in mind that you may be replacing unsightly stretch marks with unsightly scars. Otherwise simply cover them up with makeup before going to the pool or anywhere else where they will be noticed. Many types of cosmetics will hide the marks; most are creams containing masking agents such as titanium dioxide and zinc oxide. Pigments are added to provide a range of colors to match your skin's natural hue. Some good products are:

• Disappear (Ar-Ex)
• Erace (Max Factor)
• Covermark (Lydia O'Leary)
• Dermablend Cover Cream (Dermablend)

Watching weight gain during pregnancy may help control stretch marks. Unless you are overweight before pregnancy, your total weight gain should be from twenty to twenty-five pounds at a rate of two or three pounds during the first three months, then a steady gain of three-quarters of a pound a week from the fourth month on. Avoid gaining weight rapidly. Exercising to keep muscles toned will also help, as will wearing a support girdle, support pantyhose, or both.

Pregnancy and Acne

Generally skin becomes drier during the first trimester of pregnancy, then oilier toward delivery because the rise in progesterone levels causes a great increase in sebaceous activity. Among women who suffer from acne before pregnancy, it seems to clear up without treatment in 40 percent of cases, worsen in 10 percent, and stays the same in 50 percent. A small percentage of women who have never had acne may develop it during the third trimester. If you have acne during pregnancy, available treatments are very limited. Discuss your options with your dermatologist.

Other Skin and Body Changes

Half of pregnant women experience swelling of the eyelids, face, and extremities. Any moles already present may enlarge and new ones may appear. (Consult your dermatologist on the development of any new moles, as there has been an increase in the incidence of melanoma reported during pregnancy.) On the up side, common skin conditions such as psoriasis or atopic dermatitis (inherited dry skin) may improve during pregnancy.

Because of increased activity of the thyroid gland during pregnancy, you perspire more; you might also develop prickly heat. Try a stronger antiperspirant. If this doesn't work, ask your doctor to give you a prescription for the antiperspirant Dryzol.

The increased activity of the sebaceous glands at the end of pregnancy can also cause the glands of the areola to enlarge and appear as small brown elevations (called Montgomery's tubercles). These elevations can stay with you forever.

Itchy skin affects 20 percent of pregnant women. The itching, often during the third trimester, is severe and affects the entire body, although no rash accompanies it. Dry skin is caused by elevated hormonal, particularly estrogen, levels. In addition, the increase in estrogen and progesterone may lead to an improper excretion of the liver's bile acids, which collect in the bloodstream and cause the itching sensation. Try proper bathing routines for dry skin, such as oatmeal baths (see chapter 2), and use lots of moisturizers. If this doesn't clear up the problem, your doctor can give you oral antihistamines (though not all can be taken during pregnancy) and some topical steroid creams.

Genital Infections

Genital herpes is associated with specific risks during pregnancy, but only if the outbreaks appear during pregnancy. It probably increases the incidence of spontaneous abortion in early pregnancy; it may cause premature labor later in pregnancy; it definitely can infect your baby if viral shedding or outbreak occurs at the time of delivery. The incidence of baby infections is low (1 out of 3,000). If you have a history of genital herpes, your gynecologist will take cultures after the thirty-sixth week of pregnancy on a weekly basis to ensure that vaginal delivery is safe.

If you have genital warts (*condylomata acuminata*), during pregnancy they may enlarge, grow more rapidly, and increase in numbers. They may also appear for the first time during pregnancy, possibly because of the combination of increased estrogen, vascularity, and moisture. During pregnancy the usual treatment of the topical podophyllin should not be used. However, the warts can be treated surgically later in pregnancy if necessary. The presence of large warts on the vulva may indicate cesarean section. Upon delivery some of the warts will regress spontaneously.

Other infections to be aware of in relation to pregnancy:

- Vaginal moniliasis, which can be treated safely during pregnancy with miconazole (but not in the form of vaginal suppositories), Chlotrimazol, and Mycostatin (in vaginal creams or tablets)
- Trichomoniasis, which can be transmitted from infected mothers to female children
- Chlamydia trachomatis, a sexually transmitted vaginitis that can be transmitted to newborns, causing eye infections, pneumonia, and different viral infections. (Erythromycin is the treatment for pregnant women.)

Hair Changes

Unwanted Hair

Thick, lustrous, abundant hair is beautiful and a traditional sign of feminine health and sensuality. During early pregnancy the hair of the scalp usually grows vigorously, which adds to the glowing look of so many pregnant women, but just as often unwanted hair grows, primarily on the face but also on the arms and body. This usually occurs later in pregnancy because the increase in facial and body hair is related to higher progesterone levels in the body.

The unwanted facial growth can range from a light down to a heavy bristle on the skin above the upper lip and even to complete coverage on the cheeks, jaws, and chin. Many women who have never had a problem with hirsutism, the excess of hair, find they have to deal with this anguishing problem along with other difficult body changes during pregnancy.

Several standard procedures are available for dealing with excess hair, but some are not suitable for pregnant women, whose problems are generally temporary. Their hirsutism usually regresses within six months after delivery, although some women's body hair distribution may be changed permanently. (For more about coping with unwanted hair, see chapter 22.)

Thinning Hair and Postpartum Hair Loss

Few women ever go completely bald, and only a very few suffer significant hair changes with motherhood. Because women have high estrogen levels and fewer androgens in their system, they seldom get the M-shaped hairline that is so typical of male baldness (with the rare exception of some older women with lower estrogen counts). However, what seems like an incipient male patternlike baldness may appear in the final weeks of a pregnancy. This is due to a sudden drop in the estrogen level in the blood. A normal hair pattern is likely to return unaided several months after delivery.

As your body's estrogen levels rise during pregnancy, the hair of your scalp becomes softer, silkier, and glossier; hair growth phases are also longer. Because of this, more hairs than usual are in your scalp, so your hair will look and feel thicker.

Alas, in the postpartum period the luxuriant fullness of your hair is often reversed as hormone levels return to normal. Hair that would have fallen several months earlier if you weren't pregnant suddenly starts coming out. Many women seem to lose an unusual number of hairs in the weeks just after delivery and in the months following. The profuse shedding is most noticeable in front.

When the hairs do begin at last to fall, total hair volume is decreased, and the hair looks and feels thinner. A woman's normal daily hair loss of 50 to 120 hairs can double or even triple, and seeing her comb or brush laden with hair is enough to convince many a woman that she will soon be bald.

If this is happening to you, not to worry: Your hair loss is no greater than would naturally have occurred if the hair had been falling out at its normal rate over the period of months at the beginning of your pregnancy, when little hair fell away. The process is entirely reversible, even if it seems to take an eternity. If the problem bothers you a lot, your dermatologist can give you scalp lotions containing steroids or steroid injections to speed recovery (but only after delivery).

Dry Hair

Occasionally pregnant women complain of dry hair in the first trimester. Individual experience varies widely, but typically, your hair is likely to be dry for the first few months and oily for the last few months. Regular use of a protein-enriched conditioner after shampooing can do a great deal to protect each strand of hair and keep the hair smooth and glossy. Constant monitoring of your hair and scalp and changing shampoos and rinses frequently in response to the changes in your hair are recommended.

Hands and Nails

A slight flushing or reddening of the outer edges of the palms is one of the signs of pregnancy. This redness, called *palmar erythema,* continues for many women during the entire pregnancy, then disappears. It is related to increased vascular activity (an increased number of dilated blood vessels).

Your nails grow faster during pregnancy, and they can look better than ever before. Nails are structurally very much like hair: They flourish during early pregnancy because of hormonal changes within the body. Even dry, brittle nails often improve. However, also like hair, they tend to deteriorate in the first few months after the baby is born. Transverse lines and brittle and loose nails may develop.

After-Childbirth Alert

It is not frequent, but sometimes injections given as part of treatment for iron deficiency anemia, quite common following childbirth, can leave brown or blue discolorations where the needle entered the skin. These dark spots take considerable time to fade. Be sure your diet is high in iron, to avoid anemia. (See chapter 17 for more about an iron-rich diet.)

Being Beautiful—and Pregnant

Women today are usually pregnant when and because they choose to be. If you are like many expectant mothers, you have chosen the time to become pregnant because you consider yourself to be healthy and ready. During your pregnancy you probably will feel and look better than at any other time in your life.

22

THE EMBARRASSMENT
OF RICHES—
UNWANTED HAIR

Every woman wants thick, luxurious hair—on her scalp. Anywhere else it is shaved, tweezed, melted, zapped, waxed, and mercilessly rooted out. Unwanted hair is often a source of lowered self-esteem and embarrassment.

Vulnerable Areas

Hair growth is a normal bodily function. More than 25,000 hair follicles are found on the face alone, so it is not surprising that some of them are triggered into action by a variety of unexpected stimuli. Eighty-five percent of all women have hair on their arms and legs. Unwanted hair growth also frequently appears around the nipples (more rarely on the chest) and along the line extending from the navel down to the pubic hair. Tiny high-cut swimsuits make pubic hair itself a problem.

Why Hair Grows

The major factor responsible for excess hair is not the number of hair follicles, which is fixed at birth; it is the increased sensitivity of the hair follicles to the male hormones, or androgens, which can cause increased hair growth per follicle.

There are different kinds of hair on the body. Vellus hair is hardly visible.

It is short, fine, colorless, and found all over the body except for the palms and soles. Terminal hair, on the other hand, is thick and pigmented; it begins to develop at puberty. Androgens promote the conversion of vellus hairs to terminal hairs.

Your genes and the levels of stress in your life also play a role in hair growth. If your parents, siblings, aunts, uncles, and other relatives have had problems with excess hair, you probably won't be spared. Mediterranean people usually have more body hair than Orientals, for example. If your ancestors came from the Mediterranean area, you may have inherited the tendency.

Anxiety, tension, and the problems of life all conspire to affect hormone balance within the body. Stressful situations stimulate the adrenal glands to produce more androgens. This changes the body's balance of estrogen and testosterone, a male hormone which in turn can stimulate hair growth.

Many patterns of behavior lead to the production of excess adrenaline. The revved-up, overworked, type A modern woman is more likely to have problems with facial hair than her ancestors did simply because her life-style is more stimulating to the adrenal glands. Women athletes who allow their body fat to sink below 20 percent of their body weight may also find themselves strong but hairy.

Hirsutism

Hirsutism is an excessive growth of terminal hair in women, usually in the male pattern (on the upper lip, chin, sides of the cheeks, chest, abdomen, and thighs). It can also be associated with menstrual irregularities and other signs of androgen excess. Hypertrichosis, on the other hand, is a localized hair excess that is not associated with underlying endocrine problems.

If you are troubled by unwanted hair, the cause usually can be determined by consulting a physician. If your periods are irregular, see an endocrinologist or gynecologist; if they are normal, see a dermatologist.

Some disorders associated with hirsutism:

- Hypothyroidism
- Hyperthyroidism
- Anorexia nervosa
- Multiple sclerosis
- Acromegaly (enlargement of different parts of the body due to excessive secretion of growth hormone)
- Cushing's syndrome
- Insulin-resistant diabetes

Antiandrogen and Estrogen Therapy for Treating Hirsutism

Since androgens are implicated in increased hair growth and hirsutism, doctors have tried to use drugs to counter the androgen action. These drugs can be in the form of high-estrogen contraceptive pills that tip the balance of body hormones toward the feminine, or they can be in the form of antiandrogens or androgen blockers that interfere with the binding of androgens to the hair follicles. Androgen blockers cause hair to be finer and lighter and to grow more slowly in women with excessive hair growth. They also reduce the size of the oil glands (beneficial in cases of severe acne) and sometimes help reverse male-pattern baldness in women. Medications that act as androgen blockers include cyproterone acetate, which has been used successfully in Europe and Canada on many people, including male sex offenders; spironolactone (Aldactone), used primarily as a diuretic and antihypertensive, which is especially effective; and cimetidine (Tagamet), widely used for the treatment of peptic ulcers. Because one side effect of the antiandrogen drugs is a lowering of the libido (sex drive), they are seldom used. Additional side effects, particularly of cyproterone, may include dry and itching skin, depression, nausea, fatigue, increased blood pressure, and liver problems.

Medications Sometimes Linked to Unwanted Hair

Hirsutism can be a side effect of long-term administration of some medications, including:

- Androgen-dominant oral contraceptives
- ACTH and other corticosteroids
- Diazoxide (Hyperstat), used to treat elevated blood pressure
- Phenytoin (Dilantin), an anticonvulsant
- Danazol (Danocrine), a synthetic androgen used to treat fibrocystic breast disease and endometriosis
- Phenothiazines, tranquilizers
- Minoxidil (Loniten), used to treat high blood pressure

If excessive hair growth is becoming a problem for you and you are taking medication, discuss the possibility of a link with your doctor.

A woman taking antiandrogens should not get pregnant, because she runs the risk of having a feminized male offspring. Antiandrogen drug therapy is generally long-term (at least a year), with a minimum of three months necessary before any change can be expected. In many cases a combination of antiandrogens with oral contraceptives is more effective than either one alone. Contraceptives will counter the effect of excessive menstrual bleeding, a frequent side effect of antiandrogens.

Oral steroids such as low-dose dexamethazone on a daily basis are helpful in some cases of hirsutism, especially if the adrenals are overactive.

Unwanted Hair and the Aging Process

At puberty, when the adrenal cortex secretes abundant amounts of hormones, young women often notice that their eyebrows, body hair, and leg hair become thicker and darker. They may also notice a growth of downy hair on the face. In their twenties, when hormone production slows, the down on the sides of their face often disappears.

When hormone production changes, as it does during puberty, pregnancy, and menopause, the balance of estrogens and androgens changes, too. As the level of androgen increases, the growth of facial hair often increases. (In a related change, hair on the scalp may thin and male pattern baldness may begin to appear.) After menopause, the ovaries secrete very few of the estrogens that normally counterbalance the androgens in the body, and bristlelike hairs can appear on the upper lip, chin, or jaw. These hairs, which appear in 75 percent of women age sixty and older, are usually permanent.

Creams and Cosmetics

Cold cream has an undeserved reputation for stimulating the growth of facial hairs. The notion that any emollient or moisturizer can cause hair growth is incorrect. What probably gives rise to such misconceptions is that with age the skin dries and hair growth increases. Since creams are used to treat this dryness and excess hair begins to appear in the areas treated, the two are falsely associated. Another reason may be that cold cream smooths the surface of the skin, making hair more visible.

Techniques for Removing Facial and Body Hair

To remove excess hair, several standard procedures can be used. Some are more suitable for one area of the body than for another. Except for electrolysis, the effects of all methods are temporary. Cutting, shaving, waxing, applying depilatories, and tweezing do not affect the rate of hair growth or its texture.

The choice of a hair-removal method should reflect the character and amount of the hair, the area of the body where it appears, and your own personal preference. Here are the most popular methods.

Shaving

Shaving has short-lasting results, leaves blunt stubble, and is not suited for all areas of the body.

Although shaving legs, underarms, and even the bikini line usually achieves satisfactory results, shaving the face and arms is unpleasant and leaves a noticeable stubble. Contrary to what most people think, shaving does not encourage hair growth, but the emerging hair is left with blunt tips.

The result of shaving depends in good part on the quality of the tool used. If, like most women, you shave with wet hands while you are in the bath or shower, use a razor handle with a safety grip and make sure it has a fresh, good-quality blade to reduce tugging, pulling, nicks, and cuts. It is not necessary to have a new blade each time you shave, but change blades when you notice your blade getting dull (when it starts to drag along the skin). Rinse your razor thoroughly in hot water after finishing and shake it dry, but don't wipe the blade, since this will dull the shaving edge. Store the razor in a dry place so it remains clean, rust-free, and sharp.

The time you select to shave is also important. The best time to shave is not after a hair-softening soak in the tub, since long soaks result in plumped up skin, a poor surface for a really close shave. This is especially true when you plan to shave the body at the bikini line. A brief bath is all you need.

Shaving right before exposure to the sun or before swimming in a chlorine-laden pool or even salt water is also to be avoided, because these activities irritate freshly shaved skin. The best time to shave is at night.

If you shave your bikini line, you can expect the hair to grow back rapidly. The emerging bristle may rub against your thighs and irritate your skin. The solution is to shave often, even every night, during the summer season.

Never shave dry skin, because that can result in excessive pulling. Furthermore, since the hair on a woman's legs can be as tough as copper wire of the same thickness, it needs to be softened with water to make it easier to cut. Shaving creams hold moisture on the hair and also act as a lubricant. Soapsuds can do the same thing, but they are more drying, and if your area of the country has hard water, the excess calcium ions combine with soap to clog razors, so that you have to be extra careful.

For the smoothest shave, put very little pressure on the razor to avoid scraping the skin. Use long upward strokes that move against the direction of hair growth, even under the arms and other sensitive spots. With a closer shave you will shave less often.

Follow up any sort of shaving with a soothing nonalcoholic cream or lotion and a dusting powder to alleviate chafing. Do not apply a deodorant or antiperspirant directly after shaving under your arms. Shaving removes some of the outer, protective skin, and the moistness of the underarm area also sensitizes the skin. Perfumes and salts found in deodorant products can irritate vulnerable, freshly shaved skin.

Abrasives

Pumice and other abrasives have been used to rub away hair. These devices are inexpensive, easy to use, and relatively unlikely to irritate the skin—it is easy to know by discomfort when their application should be abandoned. Still, this method is not very effective and can cause irritation in some cases. The products vary from very fine sandpaper to very fine stones that are combined of pumice and other volcanic soils.

Depilatories

Depilatories chemically dissolve hair. Most commercial products remove hair easily, but they do leave a blunt stubble, as does shaving. Unfortunately, because hair and the horny layer of the epidermis are made of a similar protein substance, keratin, depilatories can be very destructive to the skin as well as to hair and cause contact dermatitis. Depilatories are highly alkaline, although many of the newer products include a skin-soothing cream or base. Most contain hydrogen sulfide, thioglycolic acid, chalk, calcium, alcohol, and sodium lauryl. They often also contain a strong perfume to counteract the unpleasant odor of hydrogen sulfide.

Depilatories are available in the form of creams, lotions, sprays, and foams. Some products that have good results and are very popular are:

- Neet (Neet Products)
- Nair (Carter-Wallace)
- Nudit (Helena Rubinstein)
- Leg Hair Remover (Scholl)

Some of these products come in lemon-scented or other scented varieties, but the scent may only add to sensitizing chemicals. Many women develop allergic reactions to the chemicals, and side effects in the form of rashes can be worse than the hair. To determine your sensitivity to these chemicals, a patch test is essential: Apply a small amount of the depilatory to the inner forearm, rinse off in ten minutes, and check the spot in twenty-four hours. If there is no reaction, go ahead and use the product.

Most important: Read the directions and use a timer. Do not allow any depilatories to remain on your skin longer than the time indicated in the directions. To remove hair on the face, be sure to use a facial depilatory.

Bleaching

Bleaching is easy to do and has fewer side effects than depilatories. For temporary growth of unwanted hair such as that experienced during pregnancy, bleaching is a good solution. The aim is to make the hair nearly invisible. Bleaching is also a good alternative for dark but fine facial hair. Any short hair (except that on the breasts, which are easily irritated) can be bleached. However, redness, mild irritation, and occasionally chemical burn can occur.

A good home bleach can be made with simple ingredients: In a glass or ceramic dish, mix together one tablespoon peroxide, one teaspoon ammonia, and one teaspoon soap suds. Apply the frothy solution to the problem area. Make sure the hairs are covered completely by the foamy suds. Allow the bleach to remain on the skin for five to ten minutes—the amount of time necessary depends on the hair color and texture. Rinse away completely with cool water and apply a moisturizer to the area. (Note: Very dark hair can acquire an orangish cast when bleached with this formula; it works best on light brown hair.)

Tweezing and Clipping

Random and unwanted hairs that appear from time to time can be clipped or tweezed. There is no evidence that plucking hairs has any effect on subsequent regrowth. It does take some time (two to four weeks) for hair to grow back. However, this method is only feasible for small areas—eyebrows, chin, areas around the nipples—and can cause ingrown hairs and folliculitis.

Waxing

Waxing any part of the body keeps hair away for about three to six weeks, but it can be painful and frequently causes ingrown hairs (especially in the bikini area). Hot wax or some other hair-capturing sticky substance is used to pull out hairs. Waxing is done professionally, but you can do it yourself. Two good waxes that are widely available are Zip Depilatory Wax (Zip) and Dorothy Gray Wax (Dorothy Gray).

Waxing is not a permanent method of hair removal, since the hair's bulb is normally not destroyed. (Bulbs may be damaged over a period of time, however, so waxing does sometimes eventually seem to lead to a thinning of the hair.) It is convenient and it gives smooth, excellent results.

Getting the Best Results from Hot Wax

Here is how to give yourself a wax treatment and get an almost professional finish:

1. Read the directions on the wax carefully so that you know exactly the temperature at which it will melt. Melt the wax in a double boiler and then remove it from the stove so that it remains at the same temperature as long as possible.
2. Dust with powder the area to be waxed.
3. Test the wax by applying it to a small area; the inside of your wrist or inner arm where there is little hair is a good place for a test. Beware of wax that is too hot: You may suffer a serious burn because it is hard to remove before it cools.
4. Spread the warm wax thickly and evenly with a wooden spatula, following the direction of hair growth.
5. Let the wax cool and harden. Apply the cloth strip firmly and pull the wax off quickly against the direction of hair growth.
6. Apply a moisturizer or anesthetic cream in a soothing base.

The danger of irritating or burning your skin with overly hot wax is minimal if you are careful to follow the product's directions exactly.

Cold Wax—The Zipping Method

Cold wax works in the same way that hot wax does. It captures the hair and then is used to pull the hair away. Many cold waxes involve the use of a cloth or fabric that is placed over the plastic wax and is used to press it around the hairs. Then it is used to pull the wax from the skin quickly and with a minimum of pain. One effective cold wax product is My-Epil (Ella Blanche).

Electrolysis

Electrolysis is the only permanent solution to unwanted hair. If the process is done correctly, hair growth is stopped because the hair bulb (follicle) is destroyed and the hair itself is removed with tweezers. Not everyone, however, is able to locate a technician with the required expertise or wishes to endure the discomfort of electrolysis or invest the time it takes. Since the method destroys one hair at a time, electrolysis is a long, often seemingly endless process. For the excessive hair growth associated with pregnancy—which often terminates during the pregnancy or soon afterward just as mysteriously as it started—electrolysis is not a logical solution. But for longer-running problems, its pros and cons are worth considering.

To destroy a hair, a skilled electrolysis operator inserts a needle into a hair follicle and transmits an electric current into the tiny hair shaft to reach the bulb at exactly the right angle to destroy it. Here is what the technician will have to be able to do:

- Locate the hair follicles
- Judge the angle at which to insert the electric needle (if the angle is wrong, pain or bleeding can result)
- Select the right amount of current
- Time the current for the exact number of seconds required

All these factors require great skill. If any one of these aspects is misjudged, the result can be disappointing: irritations, scars, and occasionally pigmentation of the skin. Even in the best hands, electrolysis is painful; your discomfort will vary depending on your own pain threshold for the area of your body involved.

The practice of electrolysis varies from state to state. Twenty-five states do not require a license for the practice of electrolysis. For this reason, competence varies a great deal. Ask your dermatologist to help you find a skilled and experienced electrologist.

The Regrowth Factor

The work of even the most skilled electrologist suffers some regrowth if the follicles have not been destroyed completely or if the hair grows at an angle, thus making it difficult or impossible to hit the germinating root. (If a follicle has been damaged but not destroyed, it can repair itself. Sometimes two follicles share the same pore and only one follicle is destroyed.) Hair on the neck often grows at an angle of about thirty degrees, whereas hair on the chin grows at about sixty degrees. If the hairs have been tweezed at all, the angle of growth may be affected, making it even more difficult to determine the exact angle of entry for the electrolysis needle. Since hairs that have been treated are always immediately plucked, it is not possible to be sure for some time whether a particular hair has been temporarily or permanently removed. Even in the best hands, about 15 to 50 percent of the hairs treated can return, requiring additional work.

The Needles Used

Two types of electrolysis needles are used. The standard fine, straight needle provides current along the entire shaft of the follicle. The newer needle is called an insulated bulbous (IB) probe; the tip directs current only on the hair follicle. This minimizes unnecessary skin damage and decreases the possibility of regrowth. Fewer retreatments are necessary and scarring is less likely. Many electrologists use both the needle and the probe, depending on the area they are treating.

After any session of electrolysis some redness is to be expected; it should disappear in a few hours. If any more serious reaction occurs, the area should be soothed with warm water compresses and over-the-counter steroid creams.

Home Electrolysis

Do-it-yourself electrolysis equipment has alternately been allowed and disallowed by the FDA. An electrolysis device requires some skill in operation. Electronic tweezers and modified forceps are also available for home use.

How to Cope with Hair Problems

Hairline.   A low forehead or a scraggly neckline can be cleaned effectively with electrolysis.

Eyebrows.   Tweezing is by far the most popular method. Although its effects are temporary, it allows a change in style that electrolysis would not.

Upper lip.   This area is popularly treated by electrolysis. It is small and progress can be seen almost immediately. The grooved area in the center of the upper lip is very sensitive and will probably require an anesthetic cream.

Jaw or chin.   Down on the side of the face can be waxed away. If the hair is coarse, electrolysis is often best. Tweezing for occasional stray hairs is also popular.

Breasts.   Small hairs around the nipples are not uncommon. They can be removed by clipping or careful plucking. A light growth of hair between your breasts can be removed by waxing or made less obvious by bleaching.

Shoulders and back. Hair in this area is usually downy. Waxing the shoulders and upper back at the beginning of the summer and then in midsummer will probably allow you to wear tanktops or other summer fashions.

Hands and arms. Bleach or wax them.

Underarms. Shaving or waxing is most usual and easy. Because of that, women seldom consider electrolysis.

Bikini area. New depilatories developed just for this area work very well, but extra caution must be taken—this area is very sensitive. If there is any stinging sensation, wash the area immediately with lukewarm water.

If you attempt to wax this area yourself, you will need patience, a good light, and a good mirror. (You will also need to be quite *agile*.) One secret to success is clipping the hair but not shaving it before you attempt to wax. Use a cold wax—it is easier to control. This is a prime area for ingrown hairs resulting from waxing.

Legs. Try bleaching for the thighs, but shaving is most popular for the legs. Waxing is okay if you are not prone to ingrown hairs.

Feet. Fret not for hairy toes. Shaving leaves a stubble; wax before you don your summer sandals.

Smooth from Top to Toe

Excessive hair growth is a problem with as many as one-third of the world's women. If you find yourself a victim, your first visit should be to your doctor and your next to the pharmacy. With knowledge, help is available.

23

ERADICATING OR MINIMIZING MOLES, MARKS, AND OTHER IMPERFECTIONS

Duringthe past year I have met with several groups of professional women to discuss skin, nail, and hair care in the context of their busy lives. Among them was an attractive banker who had perfect features, clear skin, and thick silky hair—but she also had a large mole on her neck. I found it so unbecoming that I offered to remove it for her. To my surprise, she insisted she wasn't at all bothered by it (although her hair was carefully combed to hide the blemish). Several days later she called and said, "I've been thinking. . . . I really should have that mole removed."

My banker friend now wears a short, swinging haircut; she is proud to show off her lovely neck. This charming and brilliant financial expert had probably put off having the mole removed for several years, fearing that the procedure was difficult and painful. It is a shame she waited so long.

The average human body hosts from twenty-five to fifty moles. By the time you're in your twenties, small imperfections have appeared on your skin. By the time you are sixty, spots, dots, growths, and lines decorate your skin. Every month I see dozens of patients who report vexing and unattractive marks and growths that seemed to appear overnight.

One way to preserve a youthful appearance is to keep your skin as smooth and tight as possible. Another is to keep the skin as flawless as possible—even-toned and free of marks.

Moles—Mysterious Growths

Moles (technically called nevi) are a concentration of melanocytes, the pigment or tan-producing cells in the skin. They range in color from normal flesh color to brown or bluish black. They can be raised, hairy, and rough or flat and smooth. Depending on their size and location and whether they are in clusters or alone, they can either be unattractive growths or beguiling accents for your best features.

Some moles become raised and develop a stalk or hairs; some grow larger and darker during pregnancy, puberty, when you are taking estrogen-dominant birth control pills, or after excessive sun exposure. Others disappear. If you have moles and hate them, take heart. They fade with age, and you will have fewer as you grow older. (The number of pigment cells decreases 10 to 20 percent per decade after age thirty.) In the meantime, a dermatologist can remove them.

Good Moles and Bad Moles

Exactly what causes moles is not known, but heredity and sun exposure definitely play a role. Innocent (benign) moles are rarely larger than the size of a pea, distinctly round or oval with a smooth surface, and uniform color; located on the sun-exposed parts of the body, they rarely exceed fifty in number or appear after age thirty. You should note any alteration in size, shape, color, or texture or the development of any sensation. If a mole suddenly becomes larger, darker, thicker, bleeds or crusts, or becomes itchy or painful, you should immediately consult your dermatologist—for reassurance if nothing else.

Potentially dangerous moles, called dysplastic nevi (present in about 20 million Americans), are larger than a quarter of an inch and are irregular in shape, color, and texture. They are located on the scalp, buttocks, and breasts and on the sun-exposed areas, vary from each other in appearance, are quite numerous, and keep developing after the age of thirty. To confirm the presence of a dysplastic nevus, a biopsy is essential.

The average Caucasian has an 0.5 percent chance of acquiring melanoma during his or her lifetime. For people with dysplastic moles this chance is increased tenfold. The risk is greater among those whose relatives have had melanomas.

If you have dysplastic moles, see your dermatologist regularly—at least twice a year—and keep photographs of your moles for future comparison. Avoid sun exposure (use a sunscreen with an SPF of 15) and start your children on sunscreens at six months of age whenever they go outdoors. The tendency to dysplastic moles is inherited and sunburns in childhood usually increase the risk of melanoma.

When to See a Dermatologist About a Mole

If you notice any of the following, it is wise to consult a doctor:

- Any mole that has changed in appearance
- Any new mole, especially on the palms or soles. They have increased potential for malignancy.
- Any mole that is repeatedly chafed or irritated, such as those under your bra, belt, or collar (irritation is usually due to friction)
- Any mole that shows a spread of pigmentation
- Any mole that is uncomfortable (itching, tingling, etc.)
- Any mole that you find unattractive

Turning a Liability into an Asset

Some beautiful actresses—for example, Arlene Dahl and Elizabeth Taylor—have turned moles into distinctive features. Darkening your mole or evening its color with eyebrow pencil works very well if you want to accentuate it. When you wash your makeup off, be sure to soften the color slightly with eye makeup remover or a light oil such as mineral oil before attempting to remove the makeup. Wearing the makeup does not affect the mole adversely, but rough handling may.

Congenital Moles—Birthmarks

Most moles appear after birth. About 2.5 percent of all people have birthmarks—moles present at birth. These moles are typically hairy and large, dark brown or black in color, and have a rough surface. Some, particularly those more than twenty centimeters in diameter, are called bathing trunk nevi and belong in the suspicious mole category. Fifteen percent of them undergo malignant transformation (the larger they are, the greater the malignant potential) so they should be closely watched and removed if necessary. In many cases they are removed only for cosmetic reasons.

How Your Doctor Removes a Mole

Surgically removing a mole is relatively quick and painless. The procedure is usually performed in the dermatologist's office under local anesthesia. The best cosmetic results usually are achieved with the shaving technique: The mole is shaved off with a scalpel, then an electric needle is used to electrodesiccate the base of the mole. Another technique is surgical excision followed by suturing.

Mars and Marks—Red Lines and Spots

Telangiectasia

If you are genetically disposed to it, heat, sun, cold, or even blowing your nose violently can cause some small blood vessels to lose the ability to contract. When superficial blood vessels (capillaries) become permanently dilated, they remain as tiny red or purplish lines on the face. The thinner the skin, the more apparent these so-called broken blood vessels are. Since skin becomes thinner with age, telangiectases are increasingly common after thirty. Sometimes these dilated capillaries are so numerous that the entire complexion appears flushed and ruddy.

These red lines mar the face, especially the nose and cheek areas, and may be caused by:

- Rosacea, a condition that creates dilated blood vessels
- Trauma, even a minor one such as squeezing a pimple, or rough cleansing
- Radiation, which can thin the skin
- Prolonged use of steroid creams or other steroid preparations
- Sun damage, which affects the ability of blood vessels to contract
- Hyperthyroidism
- Pregnancy and pseudopregnancy (using birth control pills)

Heredity seems to be an important factor in the appearance of these vascular blemishes, but there are certain general steps you can take to lessen the probability of developing these dilated capillaries.

If you have even one telangiectasis, these are all no-nos for you:

- Never wash with very hot or very cold water; use lukewarm water and avoid washing with hot and rinsing with cold—the change is too drastic for delicate skin.
- Avoid rough handling of skin such as with exfoliators or scrubs.
- No saunas followed by frisking in the snow—reputed to be very popular in Scandinavian countries. (Telangiectases are also common in those countries.) Again, the extremes of temperature spell trouble.
- Avoid hot and spicy foods followed by cold beverages; better still, avoid hot foods entirely.
- Don't take cold showers after exercise.
- Drink no alcohol (hot toddies are a special no-no because they are both alcoholic and served at high temperatures).
- Avoid excessive exposure to the sun and use sunscreens daily.

Erasing the Red Lines

The treatment used most often for broken capillaries is a procedure similar to electrolysis: A very fine needle is used to electrodesiccate the blood vessel. The low current causes the vessel to disappear. The larger the blood vessel, the more current is needed for good results. The number of treatments depends on the extent of the problem.

The procedure is done without anesthesia because an anesthetic might obscure the outline of the blood vessels.

Broken blood vessels are often found on the legs and are called spider veins. Heredity, long periods of standing or crossing of the legs, pregnancy or pseudopregnancy, a tendency toward varicose veins—or a combination of any of these factors and others—can be blamed. The affected veins appear as a design of threadlike bluish and purplish lines. Your dermatologist treats these by injecting a sclerosing solution into the veins. Several weeks, sometimes as long as a few months later, the blood vessels obliterate and the veins disappear.

Some doctors use an argon laser to dispatch a variety of skin blemishes. In this new technique a laser emits a blue-green light that passes harmlessly through normal skin and is eagerly absorbed by the red oxygen-carrying pigment in the blood cells. The absorbed energy is converted to heat, which cauterizes the blood vessels. Unfortunately, this treatment can result in scarring, especially on the middle face.

Age Telangiectasia

A less prevalent form of telangiectasia can also commonly be seen in women over forty. It goes by the name poikiloderma of Civatte. This condition usually involves the face, neck, and upper chest, where symmetrical netlike markings of brownish telangiectasia appear. Only the areas that have been exposed to the sun are affected; the area under the chin is usually spared. The skin becomes quite thin, with hair follicles more prominent.

Since this condition occurs mostly in women (especially those who are active outdoors), it is possible that hormones play a role in its formation. Because this condition is brought on by hormonal action combined with exposure to ultraviolet light, sunscreens should be used to avoid the problem, and bleach creams to reduce the effect.

Angiomas and Venous Lakes

Suddenly—or it seems that way—a smooth body can be dotted with tiny dome-shaped bright red lesions. Because of their color, these are called cherry or ruby angiomas. These marks have no malignant potential and are not dangerous. They are primarily a cosmetic problem, more common in aging women or men. They usually appear on the trunk and upper thighs, rarely on the face. The treatment of these tiny red bumps is simple: a touch-up with an electric needle.

Venous lakes are dilated veins found on sun-exposed areas. The treatment is similar to that for cherry angiomas.

Those Awful Marks—Brown Spots and Growths

Age spots (lentigines). Age spots, also called liver spots, have nothing to do with the liver. Nor are they ordinary freckles. They are a sign of age and a sign you don't want. Unlike freckles, liver spots do not fade in winter. They may appear singly and are larger in size than a freckle. Developing from about the age of thirty onward and seen initially on the face and later on hands, wrists, and forearms, these flat, round, or oval marks are light brown or tan (with time they turn dark brown) and have distinct, irregular edges. They have no texture; all of a sudden they just show up, making you feel speckled and old. They represent the cumulative effect of years of sun exposure.

Porcelain spots. A condition usually seen in women over thirty, these white spots appear on the legs and arms, particularly on sun-exposed areas such as hands and forearms, and represent a local decrease in pigment production. The condition is not associated with any symptoms; it simply indicates sun damage and can tell others a little bit about your age. Unfortunately, there is no treatment except camouflaging the spots with makeup.

Sebaceous gland hyperplasias. These lesions are very common, especially after the age of forty. They usually appear on the forehead, cheeks, and nose as yellowish bumps with a central indentation. Such bumps can be treated with electrodesiccation, cryosurgery, trichloroacetic acid, or Accutane.

Milia. This affliction, too, is more common among mature women. Milia are the white minicysts that appear on the face, particularly around the eyes and on the eyelids. These mars resemble whiteheads and may be numerous. The use of occlusive, greasy cosmetics (such as some eye creams), sun exposure, and heredity are factors that can predispose skin to milia. They are usually treated by a dermatologist by pricking and then draining them (as with whiteheads). Electrodesiccation can be used in some cases to remove them.

Seborrheic keratoses. Pigmented brown to black growths that resemble warts may be keratoses. They can appear on the body as well as the face, neck, and extremities; may be single or multiple; and are particularly common in the over-forty age group. They are usually slow-growing. Happily, they are neither potentially malignant nor contagious. However, the sudden appearance of many may herald an underlying problem and you should consult your doctor. As with many skin conditions, heredity plays a part.

If the keratoses makes you feel uncomfortable or unattractive, they can be removed by scraping (curettage), electrically burning (electrodesiccation), or freezing (cryosurgery). In some cases multiple keratoses that are shallow, usually found on the lower extremities (stucco keratoses), can be treated nonsurgically with a prescription moisturizing agent (Lac-Hydrin Lotion/Westwood, for example).

Getting Rid of Mars and Marks

Bleach Creams

Hormonal imbalances during pregnancy, rubbing your skin, industrial chemicals, exposure to the sun, and a host of other environmental factors can darken areas on your skin. Uneven color and discoloration is not always attributable to age, but age is a factor.

Bleaches do not actually change the color of the skin. Rather, they prevent melanin formation. A variety of different substances have been used to bleach the skin: lemon juice, tea, even salicylic acid. Ammoniated mercury was used until 1974, when it was barred by the FDA because of its toxicity and the incidence of allergic reactions. The best lightening agent now in use is hydroquinone. Concentrations of more than 2 percent have to be prescribed by a doctor and are available in a variety of creams, gels, and solutions. Many of these preparations also include other substances to soothe skin and emollients to protect skin; most include a sunscreen or sunblock. As a rule, over-the-counter preparations are ineffective because concentrations of hydroquinone are inadequate.

Exactly how hydroquinone fades skin spots remains unclear. Most scientists believe the compound inhibits the enzyme tyrosinaze, essential in melanin formation. However, hydroquinone bleach preparations are actually only partially effective, lightening dark spots about 50 percent and working most satisfactorily on relatively light spots. In addition, these bleaching agents work very slowly.

Don't use any bleach preparation without trying a patch test on your inner arm first to check for allergic reaction. Also be aware that any exposure to the sun will encourage the bleached areas to darken again.

One very effective commercial product is the prescription drug Melanex Solution (Neutrogena), but it does not contain sunscreen, so additional protection is a must. Two bleaching products containing 4 percent hydroquinone (available by prescription only):

- Solaquin Forte Cream and Gel (Elder)—cream for dry skin, gel for oily
- Eldopaque Forte Cream (Elder)—offers the highest amount of protection; good for use after chemical peeling or during pregnancy

Peeling the Spots

For fast, sure results, chemical peeling is quite effective. The procedure is done by a dermatologist. Trichloroacetic acid is applied to spots in varying concentrations depending on the color of the spots. The technique works better on the face than on other parts of the body.

After peeling it is mandatory that you avoid the sun and use sunblock; sun exposure could make age spots reappear. (See chapter 8 for more on peels.)

Other Treatments

Electrodesiccation (burning the spot with an electric needle) and cryosurgery (freezing) can also be used. Again, sun exposure after treatment will cause spots to reappear.

Flawless Beauty

We all admire the smooth, perfect skin of youth. It can be yours for years longer if you avoid abusing your skin—and if you consider small repairs to your face, such as ridding yourself of broken capillaries—a part of your regular health program. It is not vanity; it is self-protection.

24

GLOW AND
STAY DRY

When I get stuck in traffic, wear heavy clothing, play tennis, or speak at conferences, I perspire. I know it is a normal function, but it is irritating and uncomfortable. While there appears to be no perfect solution, some methods will work to help you "keep cool" (and dry).

Perspiration is a natural mechanism the body uses to regulate its temperature and, to a lesser degree, rid itself of wastes. When you are subjected to heat—as when you are in a cramped, overheated car or commuter train—your internal temperature rises. Internal heat dilates the blood vessels and forces more blood to the surface of your skin for cooling. Your skin becomes pink, rosy, and flushed, exactly as it does when you have a fever.

At the same time, your brain signals 2 million or more sweat glands in your body to flood your skin with watery perspiration. These millions of glands can collectively produce about a quart of perspiration on an average day, somewhat less on a cool, inactive day, and more than twice as much on a warm, tense, busy day. When air passes over the perspiration-moist skin, convection (the transfer of heat via movement of the air) increases, and so does evaporation, cooling your skin and body.

Your body releases about 600 calories of heat in one quart of perspiration. Sweat is naturally produced at a "resting" temperature of about 88°F, but with exercise, perspiration can be produced at any temperature. We all perspire all the time—even during sleep.

Where Does Sweat Come From?

Sweat is the secretion of two types of glands: the eccrine glands and the apocrine glands. The eccrine glands are responsible for most wetness; the apocrine glands are responsible for the secretions that provide food for the bacteria that cause body odor.

Eccrine glands are located in tiny wells that are independent of hair follicles; they originate directly from the epidermis and are widely distributed over the body. They are most numerous on the palms and the soles, with an ample number on the forehead. This accounts for sticky palms and moist feet (on a normal day of walking, feet can produce as much as a quarter of a cup of perspiration) and for dripping foreheads. Perspiration glands are least numerous on your arms and legs. Because these glands help prevent skin dryness, your arms and legs tend to be drier than other parts of the body.

Apocrine glands are larger in size but fewer in number than the eccrine glands and are restricted to the armpits (axillae), anogenital region, areolae (the areas around the nipples), the external ear canal (glands that produce ear wax), eyelids, and around the belly button. The apocrine glands, like oil glands, terminate in hair follicles.

Apocrine gland development is regulated by sex hormones that become active at puberty and decrease markedly in old age. Without the stimulation of the sex hormones, there is little apocrine perspiration. This is why prepubescent children and elderly people do not usually suffer from body odor.

A sweat gland usually is a corkscrew-shaped tube that starts in the lower level of the skin (the dermis) and winds up to the surface of the skin. It finally emerges on the surface of your skin through a sweat pore, not visible to the naked eye.

What Is Perspiration Made Of?

Eccrine sweat is a colorless, odorless solution composed of 99 percent water. The remaining 1 percent of eccrine perspiration is made of:

Salt	Chloride	Urea	Protein
Amino acids	Calcium	Potassium	Iron
Lactate	Glucose	Phosphorus	Lipids

This perspiration is actually very similar to weak urine. Some medical scientists believe that eccrine perspiration contributes to healthy kidney function, because the more perspiration produced, the less waste the kidneys have to process. This can be beneficial for sports or other activities that put stress on the bladder. Perspiration is important to your total body health.

Apocrine sweat is milky, scant, and slightly yellowish in color. It is produced in tiny droplets at irregular intervals, and the droplets dry to sticky granules that adhere to the hairs and clothing. The perspiration produced contains short-chain fatty acids and sulphurated protein by-products—a virtual banquet for bacteria. It is the action of the bacteria on the perspiration that causes odor.

Two modes of attack are used to avoid body odor:

1. Reducing wetness with an antiperspirant
2. Reducing bacteria with a deodorant

Who Perspires Most, Men or Women?

Men and women perspire differently. Women produce less sweat per gland, while men produce approximately one-third more. Perhaps that is the reason that women often glow with an all-over moisture while men very obviously perspire. It may be that men produce more perspiration simply because they are usually larger and so have more body surface.

Sweat concentration varies from person to person. Heavy, large people of both sexes seem to sweat more: The more surface, the more perspiration; the more perspiration, the more chance of body odor. The number of apocrine glands also varies: They are most numerous in persons of African descent, less numerous in Caucasians, and least numerous in Orientals.

A woman's sweat pH is in the acid range, between 4.5 and 5.5. The more slowly you sweat, the lower the pH. Thus, as you exercise or are more active, you sweat more quickly and alter this chemical composition. A woman who exercises will produce a more concentrated sweat (with a pH up to 6.5) than a sedentary woman and needs to be more careful about the deodorant/antiperspirant products she uses. Such concentrated sweat becomes a breeding ground for bacteria, and the faster you sweat the stronger the odor. So when you are active be sure to use a deodorant as well as an antiperspirant.

Advertising often plays on the fact that women seem to be more sensitive to odor, while men are more sensitive to wetness. Women tend to use more deodorants and antiperspirants than needed. For maximum security, combine the blocking ingredients of an antiperspirant with the bacteria-fighting ingredients of a deodorant. Any product that makes you feel more secure may also help control perspiration because you know that you are prepared and can relax.

The Mystery of How to Stop Perspiration

In order to be considered a true antiperspirant, a product must reduce perspiration by at least 25 percent. Exactly how antiperspirants work is not known. It is believed that chemical salts react with a protein to form an insoluble salt at the orifice of the sweat gland on the skin's surface. The salt forms a plug, preventing perspiration from escaping the duct. Because plugging the pores affects body function, antiperspirants are considered drugs by the FDA. Deodorants work on the surface of the skin to fight odor. Since they do not affect body functions in any way, they are classified by the FDA as cosmetics.

Most of the chemicals that retard the flow of sweat are based on astringent salts. The most popular astringent salts are:

Aluminum chlorohydrate	Zinc phenolsulfonate
Aluminum phenolsulfonate	Aluminum sulfate
Zirconyl chloride	Zirconium chlorohydrate
Aluminum chloride	

Whether you buy pads, creams, sprays, sticks, lotions, powders, liquids, roll-ons, or aerosols, antiperspirants rely on similar chemical formulas designed to prevent moisture release. Each type of product has its following; however, some types are demonstrably more effective than others:

Type of Product	Effectiveness
Liquids and aerosols	20 percent
Sticks, lotions, creams	40 percent
Roll-ons	50 percent

Occasionally people experience a reaction to inhaling spray from aerosol cans; incidents of lung damage from this source have been recorded. If you use an aerosol, be sure you carefully direct spray away from your face.

For some people, too much sweating causes breakouts because sweat can be occlusive. You can avoid blemishes by using antiseptic astringents—Sebanil (Owen), for example. Blot often to avoid perspiration buildup on the surface. Carry Buf-Puf Singles (Personal Care Products/3M) to clear perspiration on the face.

When and How to Apply an Antiperspirant

If you are concerned about underarm wetness, you probably prefer an antiperspirant to a deodorant. Don't apply antiperspirant while you are perspiring or after a shower—the active chemicals will not penetrate the skin effectively or may be too irritating. It is best to apply an antiperspirant at night before bed. The antiperspirant affects your pore openings during the night and you will be protected from wetness the following morning. If you shower in the morning, wait until your underarms are completely dry before applying antiperspirant.

Several months ago a young systems analyst who often travels for business came to me with a perspiration problem. Her blouse was soaked; even the bulky pads she wore under her arms were soggy. Her problem was affecting her job performance and career as well as her personal life. I gave her the prescription antiperspirant Drysol (Person & Covey) and a list of guidelines that have kept her more dry and less worried than before.

Six Tips for Effective, Nonirritating Antiperspirant Use

1. Restrict the application of the antiperspirant to the vault or top of the armpit. This limits the area that can be adversely affected and concentrates the antiperspirant where it is most needed.
2. Stop using a product if you begin to experience itching, tingling, or stinging or if you develop any redness in the underarm area.
3. Don't apply an antiperspirant on broken or irritated skin or use one immediately after shaving or showering.
4. Hair-free underarms reduce the likelihood of odor.
5. If you use a spray or aerosol, hold the container at least six inches from the underarm area and avert your head to avoid breathing the fumes.
6. Rub the product in with your fingers for best results.

If you want instant action, use a roll-on, because it applies antiperspirant ingredients most directly to the underarms. Sticks and aerosols are less effective because antiperspirant salts must be dissolved before they can work. Antiperspirants have a cumulative effect: If you use a product consistently, you can safely skip a day or two, unless you will be under exceptional emotional stress.

Antiperspirants will not completely stop the flow of perspiration, which is good, since the secretion of sweat is essential to the regulation of the body's temperature and water metabolism. Antiperspirant fade-out is due to the fact that many antiperspirants limit perspiration only a little. When you are very active or very hot, you perspire so much that a weak antiperspirant has little value. (Adding more of the same antiperspirant won't help much because the heavy flow of perspiration washes away the chemicals before they have a chance to work.)

In severe cases of excessive perspiration, Drysol (Person & Covey), a prescription solution containing aluminum chloride in alcohol, is remarkably effective in reducing underarm, palm, and foot sweating.

Fighting Odor

If odor is a problem, the following suggestions will keep you fairly dry and odor-free:

• Wash at least once a day, and use a deodorant soap under the arms and in the groin. (Never use a deodorant soap on your face. Many include

antibacterial chemicals that may invite photosensitive reactions mani-
festing as rashes when your skin is exposed to light.)
- Keep your feet, underarms, and unexposed parts of the body dry at all times.
- Wear absorbent 100 percent cotton underwear, and change it often.
- Avoid tight and plastic or rubber shoes and boots.
- Use absorbent deodorant powders: on your feet for foot odor, in your bra for body odor (especially if you have heavy breasts), and on your palms for sticky hand syndrome. Try Formula Magic (Consolidated Chemical) or Lobana Body Powder (Ulmer).

The tendency to perspire heavily seems to run in families.

If you have to worry about perspiration when you dress in the morning, both your wardrobe and your emotional life are subjected to strain. You will feel better if you take some action, even with simple home remedies.

New and Dry Methods of Odor Fighting

Many early deodorants were simply perfumed alcohols that masked the unpleasant odors caused by bacteria. Modern deodorant compounds work by reducing or eliminating the offending bacteria. Newer preparations usually rely on antibacterial agents such as neomycin, triclosan, and phenyl-mercuric nitrate held in liquids or soaps to destroy the odor-creating organisms. For persons allergic to these chemicals in popular commercial deodorants, hypoallergenic products that contain quaternary ammonium or chlorhexidine compounds are available.

A relatively new ingredient in deodorants, cyclomethicone, causes liquids on the skin to evaporate. The evaporation is so rapid that the products feel dry, without any oily sensation, on application. Some of the products that include this feature are:

- Secret Antiperspirant (Procter & Gamble)
- Arrid Extra Dry (Carter)
- Mitchum (Mitchum)
- Sure (National)

Occasionally people do suffer reactions from commercially prepared deodorants. If an allergic reaction or irritation has been your experience, stop using the offending product and try one or a combination of these home products: plain baking soda, baby powder, talcum powder.

Soaps and Perfumes

Soaps advertised as deodorant soaps work by washing away bacteria from the surface of your body and leaving a residue of antibacterial chemicals, usually combined with a floral-, lemon-, or pine-scented perfume. Deodorants containing fragrances can cause allergic reactions. Any of them can also produce an irritant dermatitis, especially right after shaving or bathing, because the chemicals used, especially salts, are irritants. (For more about chemicals that cause irritation and allergic reaction, see chapter 19.)

Perfumed deodorants and body sprays combining a mild deodorant with a delicately scented cologne can be used as all-over body refreshers. Examples of these products are:

- Impulse Body Spray (Lever Brothers)
- Musk Jasmine Perfume Deodorant Body Spray (Love)
- Energizing Body Spray (Jean Naté)

Keeping Hands and Feet Odor Free

Do your palms get hot and damp or cold and clammy? Just fan your hands through the air for instant relief. If the problem is persistent, keep a supply of talcum powder, cologne, or witch hazel with you and apply it when the need and opportunity arise. Wash your hands often with cool tap water, and after they are patted dry, apply an antiperspirant to your palms.

The prescription antiperspirant Drysol can also be used for excessive perspiration of the hands.

1. Just before retiring, dry your palms with a towel and apply Drysol. (Do not wash your hands before application.)
2. Cover your palms with clear plastic wraps (use Saran Wrap), and cover with gloves to hold the wraps in place.
3. Now off to bed. In the morning remove the coverings and wash your hands.

Repeat this procedure nightly for about three or four weeks. A maintenance program of about once a week should be sufficient from then on.

A household remedy that works very well for controlling moist palms and smelly feet is soaking in strong tea. Use tea soaks once or twice daily at first; after the problem is under control, use them biweekly for maintenance.

1. Boil several tea bags in one quart of water for about ten minutes.
2. Add enough cold water to make a comfortable soak.
3. Soak hands or feet for twenty to thirty minutes.
4. Dry and apply a light talc or powder.

Be careful not to get hands or feet so dry that the skin cracks.

Hyperhidrosis

About one person in ten has overactive eccrine glands. Excessive sweating is called hyperhidrosis. It can occur in perfectly normal, healthy women and even in children; it is often a response to stress. People who suffer from obesity, diabetes, thyroid problems, or certain neurologic disorders are more prone to hyperhidrosis. Some medications such as the beta-blocker propranolol may cause profuse generalized sweating.

Generalized hyperhidrosis also accompanies fever. Most hyperhidrosis is emotionally induced and localized in the palms, soles, and armpits. Cold injury and early rheumatoid arthritis may be associated with localized hyperhidrosis.

Some treatment suggestions:

- Change socks or stockings twice daily.
- Cleanse the feet nightly with Dr. Scholl's Granulated Foot Soap.
- Soak the feet in Burow's solution nightly.
- Avoid rubber- or plastic-soled shoes.
- Apply a lotion of 10 percent tannic acid and 70 percent alcohol every morning and every evening. (Ask your pharmacist to prepare a half pint of the formula, enough to last several weeks.)

Both the doctor and the patient must be alert to allergic reactions to any of the products.

Sweat leaches out chemicals called chromates, used in leather dyes. A reaction to chromates is sometimes partly responsible for irritations of the feet, so controlling perspiration is essential. Avoid high shoes, boots, and cordovan-tanned leathers in unlined shoes. Zeasorb Powder (Stiefel) and Breezee Mist Foot Powder (Pedinol) are excellent products that have helped many of the afflicted.

Iontophoresis Apparatus

The word *iontophoresis* means the transfer of ions, or electrically charged atoms, usually with the creation of an electric field. The usual iontophoresis apparatus is an electric battery device that seems to stop perspiration. Several attachments are available, specifically shaped for the feet, hands, and armpits. When a mild charge is delivered by the machine, the salt molecules of the perspiration glands are affected, and the treated area remains dry for approximately six to eight weeks. The device, available with a prescription, can be used at home. Four to six weekly treatments of fifteen to twenty minutes each are usually needed after an initial seven to ten days of daily treatments.

Other Antihyperhidrosis Methods

For all-over hyperhidrosis, oral prescription medications are available. These include:

- Tranquilizers (if the hyperhidrosis is stress induced) such as Valium (diazepam)
- Anticholinergic agents (the Banthine/Pro-Banthine group, Pamine, Robinul), particularly when taken just before a stressful situation
- Indomethacin (usually used for arthritis)

The problem with most of these medications, however, is that the doses required to inhibit excessive sweating also inhibit the secretion of saliva, thus causing dry mouth and gastrointestinal problems. Also, such medications cannot be used by those with severe bowel disease or glaucoma.

In very severe cases of palmar hyperhidrosis (excessive sweating of the palms), a cervical sympathectomy, or severing of the nerves associated with the sweating of the palms, can be performed. This surgery usually reduces perspiration about 50 to 80 percent. Removal of sweat glands may be done on the vault of the armpit or other small areas that produce high volumes of perspiration. This operation should be considered only as a last resort.

Food, Medicine, and Odor

People with problems of heavy apocrine perspiration and bromhidrosis (body odor) should avoid certain foods that, when carried through the bloodstream and body fluids, tend to be excreted with sweat and create body odor. These foods are:

Garlic	Mustard	Beer (and many other
Onions	Vinegar	alcoholic beverages)
Hot spices	Sharp cheeses	

Excessive localized perspiration may result after eating spicy food, peanut butter, coffee, chocolate, and foods containing citric acid. Those with sweaty palms should avoid eggs, liver, and other foods that contain lecithin. Chronic alcoholics are prone to body odors. The vast majority of bromhidrosis sufferers have inherited the tendency. (For more on odor-making foods, see chapter 17.)

Hot Flashes

Perspiring freely makes you more prone to possible odor. Menopausal women often suffer from what are known as hot flashes—a sudden feeling of warmth on the upper body, especially the shoulders, neck, back, and upper arms. This uncomfortable sensation is followed by profuse perspiration that leaves a cold and clammy sensation and a feeling of exhaustion.

Flashes usually appear about the time of the cessation of menstruation, although they are not necessarily triggered by estrogen levels. Many women who suffer flashes find that their only help is a strong deodorant and wearing layered garments that can be removed quickly and easily when a flash is coming on. Avoiding warm environments such as overheated rooms is helpful.

Night Sweats

Another problem of women over forty is night sweats. The victim awakes from sleep drenched in perspiration and feels stifled by the heat. Like fever, night sweats can be a symptom of a more serious problem. They were once associated with tuberculosis, but they can be a symptom of chronic infection, an undetected malignancy, or a metabolic disorder. Be very wary of a sudden occurrence and check with your physician.

Heat Rashes

Prickly heat is an itchy rash caused by sweat retention due to a temporary blockage of the sweat ducts and sweat pores. When perspiration is blocked from reaching the skin's surface, the force of the entrapped liquid may break through the walls of the sweat ducts and create an inflammatory reaction. It can be caused by wearing plasticized or rubber clothing that doesn't allow for the absorption or evaporation of perspiration. For example, a plastic belt can lead to a heat rash under the belt. The rash can also occur as a result of prolonged bathing, excessive exercise, sunburn, or during a febrile illness.

Prickly heat is very common in infants, who suffer from itchy pinhead-sized pimples. It can be a problem for runners who perspire profusely and for anyone who wears a heavy rubber or plastic sweatsuit that holds body moisture in. Other victims include heavy women and women with large breasts or soft body folds that retain moisture. Don't allow perspiration moisture to remain on your body; wash as soon as possible and dry completely.

Some heat rash soothers:

- Refrigerated light moisturizing lotion, such as Keri Light (Westwood) or Nutraderm (Owen)
- Cool, wet compresses
- For itchiness, an over-the-counter anesthetic preparation such as Prax Lotion (Ferndale)
- Absorbent powders
- One gram of vitamin C taken daily to alleviate the fatigue that commonly accompanies an outbreak of prickly heat

A Word on Saunas and Steam Baths

One method of inducing perspiration is the sauna. A sauna exposes the body to high temperatures in order to bring on profuse perspiration. It shocks the body and often doubles the heart rate. Dehydration is never good for the skin, and for many people, saunas involve a trade-off: five pounds of temporary weight loss in exchange for dry, parched skin. Saunas can also be a health hazard for those with high blood pressure. (True, saunas have long been popular in Scandinavian countries, but remember that people there use saunas throughout their lives, so their bodies learn to accommodate to rapid heating when they are young. The sauna in Scandinavia is considered a method of cleansing and relaxing the body, not just a means to reduce weight.)

If you enjoy basking in heat and perspiring freely, choose a steam bath over a sauna. But avoid both if you have a tendency to broken capillaries or acne rosacea.

Keeping Sweet

Cool showers, light and loose-fitting clothing, careful drying, dusting with powders, and the use of body sprays can all help you stay sweet. They cut the chances of your skin being attacked by microorganisms and encourage the calm that can help cut excessive perspiration and diminish body odor. If you exercise—and you should—be sure to wash carefully after each exercise session. Washing will rid the skin of dried perspiration residue, keep the pores open, and reduce odor.

Keep your exercise clothes very clean. The best method of controlling any type of body odor is through personal cleanliness: frequent bathing and thorough cleaning and laundering.

However anxiety-inducing the situation or hot the temperature, fretting about sweating doesn't do much good, and it can make things worse. Perspiration helps your body to function; be thankful for it.

25

BEHAVIOR THAT
WRECKS
YOUR LOOKS

Drug abuse is everywhere. The signs are visible to anyone who pays attention to herself and to others. I have patients who come in for a minor skin problem, and after I look at them, I say to myself, "This woman has been drinking (or taking drugs) for a long time." It makes me sad, because my patient is involved in behavior that is harming her body and her skin. Some of the most destructive addictions start as habits. The trick is to stop them—immediately—before they affect your looks and your life.

Cigarettes

When you smoke you are taking risks: Chances of developing lung cancer are twenty times greater than for nonsmokers, and there is an increased susceptibility to cancer of the bladder, mouth, larynx, and pancreas.

Dermatologists have long noticed that women who smoke are more apt to develop fine lines and wrinkles, especially around the eyes and mouth. I have seen the difference in my own patients. The wrinkling is due to the vascular constricting effect of nicotine, which results in a curtailed blood supply. Another possible explanation is that each time she draws on a cigarette, a smoker must use her facial muscles, puckering her lips and squinting her eyes. A one-pack-a-day smoker repeats that action about 70,000 times a year. These two factors alone may cause skin to age faster.

But other factors usually come into play as well—sun exposure, for example. The combination of smoking and sun exposure doubles the damage to skin.

Dr. Thomas Rees, a noted plastic surgeon, found that smoking has a noticeable impact on healing following cosmetic surgery. Because nicotine constricts blood vessels, patients who smoked healed more slowly than others.

In addition, people who smoke have a larger number of yellowish bumps (sebaceous gland hyperplasia) on the face, and they may also experience greater hair loss than nonsmokers.

Sleeping Pills

Sleeping pills often contain barbiturates that can affect the skin. One of the most commonly used barbiturates, phenobarbital, can be responsible for new acne lesions or the aggravation of existing ones.

Sometimes a red rash appears on the face and upper part of the body a few days after a barbiturate is taken. Barbiturates can also cause a condition called fixed drug eruption in which a round red or purple lesion on the skin recurs with each barbiturate intake and leaves a permanent brownish discoloration.

In some cases, barbiturates have been known to cause widespread shedding of the epidermis, a very serious condition requiring hospitalization, as well as barbiturate pressure blisters at pressure points of the body such as the ankles, heels, and hips.

Caffeine

Caffeine belongs to the family of chemicals known as methylxanthines, found in more than sixty different kinds of plants. The most common sources of methylxanthines are coffee and cocoa beans, tea leaves, and cola nuts.

Caffeine exacerbates many problems: It aggravates dryness and makes itches itchier and jitters worse; it can help migraine headaches, but it can also trigger them. Like nicotine, caffeine is a vasoconstrictor, diminishing the blood supply to the skin.

The caffeine/sleeplessness cycle that is so easily set up by modern lifestyles can end in a skin-dulling (and mind-dulling) pattern. Coffee, tea, cocoa, cola, chocolate, and many over-the-counter medications keep the level of caffeine in your blood high during the day. The effect of caffeine can last up to twenty hours.

Instant coffee has less caffeine than brewed coffee, and decaffeinated coffee still less, but fruit juices, herbal teas, and water have none at all.

Marijuana

THC (tetrahydrocannabinol), the active ingredient in marijuana, is absorbed into the bloodstream if it is smoked or eaten in foods. Marijuana can aggravate acne and accelerate hair loss in addition to disturbing several physiological functions.

Cocaine

Because, like nicotine and caffeine, cocaine is a vasoconstrictor and slows blood circulation, it may follow that the skin reacts in the same way as it does to nicotine. The slower the circulation, the less blood can flow through the skin's blood vessels. Since the healthy pink coloration of the skin is due in large part to the color of the blood circulating under the skin's surface, less blood circulation means less of this pink color and a more sallow, tired-looking skin.

Alcohol

A little wine with your dinner or even one martini does not harm your complexion. There is some evidence that it might even improve your heart function by slightly dilating the blood vessels. Anything more than that, even moderate drinking, can be damaging: The dilated blood vessels weaken. With age, the tiny blood vessels no longer contract normally but are seen as small red lines on the face and body (telangiectasia). Sometimes these lines appear in the shape of a spider (spider angioma).

People who drink, especially beer and sherry lovers, have an increased incidence of rosacea as a result of the vasoactive chemicals tyramine and histamine, which cause facial flushing. Alcohol flush becomes more prominent in combination with some medications—antidiabetic drugs such as chlorpropamide, antifungal drugs such as griseofulvin, and antibiotics such as cephalosporins. Chemicals present in mushrooms also aggravate alcohol flush. (For more information on rosacea, see chapter 5.)

Other skin conditions triggered or aggravated by alcohol consumption include:

- Hives
- Psoriasis
- Dandruff
- Fungal infections
- Nummular eczema, which appears as coin-shaped, itchy, red scaly patches usually found on the extremities

Alcohol is a dehydrator; it steals water from your skin. If you are thirsty the morning after drinking more than your quota, you should realize that your skin is dry and thirsty also. The alcohol leaches water from the tissues and depletes the vitamin C levels, making skin flaky and dull. It is very important to replace the water you lose after drinking. Drink fluids such as water and citrus juice and steam your skin lightly to rehydrate it.

Alcohol also interferes with the absorption of calcium and may be linked with osteoporosis.

Other Drugs

Amyl and butyl nitrites. Found in glue, correction fluid, paint thinner, and other toxic materials, these chemicals irritate the nose so much that the skin may peel constantly. The fumes from these poisons interfere with the body's ability to obtain oxygen and may make the skin look slightly blue and sickish. Lack of oxygen slows cell growth. If liquid nitrite touches the skin, a chemical burn may appear (this is more common in smokers because nitrites are flammable). Those who use nitrites have been known to be at higher risk of contracting AIDS (acquired immune deficiency syndrome), possibly because nitrite usage relaxes the anal sphincter, thus causing an easier transmission of the virus during anal intercourse.

Amphetamines. These stimulants of the central nervous system, sometimes found in diet pills or stay-awake products, can cause itchy rashes or asthma attacks. Even in low doses these drugs make the mouth and lips very dry. People who use them habitually lick their lips, causing severe chapping. Amphetamines may also cause increased hair loss and sweating.

Heroin. Heroin can destroy your looks. The areas where drugs are injected become scarred and the veins become clogged with blood clots. Ulcers, discolorations, infections, blisters, and abscesses can develop. In addition, heroin slows all body functions, including the regeneration of skin cells. Most heroin addicts look years older than they are and fall victim to severe yeast infections of the skin and other organs of the body.

It's in Your Power

Age, environment, genes, and to some extent life-style and stress are all problems over which you have limited control. The use of drugs and the skin problems they inspire, however, are entirely in your power to control or avoid.

CONCLUSION

I hope that this book has answered some of your questions and dispelled some of the mystery around skin care. Perhaps the next time you travel, try a new sport, or just want to choose a new shampoo, it can serve you as a guide.

Finally, I hope that the years will always show in your wisdom, not on your skin.

INDEX

Perspiration, 271
applying antiperspirant, 274–275
composition of, 272–273
fighting odor in, 275–277
foods that tend to stimulate odor in, 213
and heat rashes, 280
and hot flashes, 279
and hyperhidrosis, 277–279
and night sweats, 279–280
origin of sweat, 272
sexual differences in, 273
stopping, 273–274
Petroleum jelly, and lip protection, 114
Phenobarbital, and acne, 29
Phenol, 85
Phenothiazines, lip problems from, 115
Phenytoin, and acne, 29
PHISO AC BP Cream (Winthrop Breon), 33
Phosphorus, 203
Photosensitizing foods, 213
Picture Perfect Color Rinse (Clairol), 172
Pill acne, 230
Piz Buin 8 (Greiter), 56
Piz Buin 8 or 15 (Greiter), 58
Piz Buin Stick (Greiter), 113
Plantar calluses, 138
Plantar warts, 139–140
Plants, and contact dermatitis, 228
Poison ivy, 132–133
Polysporin Ointment (Burroughs Wellcome), 118
Polysporin Powder (Burroughs Wellcome), 130
Polysporin Spray (Burroughs Wellcome), 130
Polytar (Stiefel), 157
Porcelain Cover Base (Adrien Arpel), 87
Porcelain spots, 268
Porcelana (Jeffrey Martin), 72
Pore lotion, 92
Pore Minimizer (Clinique), 45

Pore Minimizer Makeup (Clinique), 94
Pores, cleaning of, 25–26
Postpartum alopecia, 165–166
Potassium, 204
Powder, 97–98
finding right shade of, 98
Prax Cream and Lotion (Ferndale), 132
Prax Lotion (Ferndale), 60, 280
Preference (L'Oréal), 173
Pregnancy
and acne, 249
and broken blood vessels, 245–246
and changes in hands and nails, 252
and changes in skin color, 243–245
and genital infections, 250
and hair changes, 251–252
and hormonal changes, 242–243
and itchy skin, 250
and moles, 249
and Montgomery's tubercles, 250
and mottled skin, 247
and prickly heat, 249–250
and skin tags, 248
and stretch marks, 248–249
and varicose veins, 246–247
Premalignant lesions, 62
Premiere Perm (L'Oréal), 180
Presoaping, 25
Presun 15 Ultra Sunscreen Lip Protector (Westwood), 113
Presun 15 (Westwood), 56, 57
Presun Facial Sunscreen (Westwood), 56
Prickly heat, 249–250, 280
Progesterone
and acne, 28
levels of, during pregnancy, 242–243
Prosaglandins, 60
Protein, 201
Protein Color Rinse (Nestlé), 172
Protein Pac Treatment (Vidal Sassoon), 153
P & S (Baker/Cummins), 158
Psoriasis, 193, 284